The Single Woman's Guide to a Happy Pregnancy

Fourth Edition

Mari Gallion

Copyright © 2016 Mari Gallion

All rights reserved.

ISBN: 1539049612

ISBN 13: 9781539049616

Table of Contents

Preface		v
Introduction		vii
Chapter One	This Was My Wake-up Call	1
Chapter Two	Banishing the Negative, Cherishing the Positive	11
Chapter Three	Life Starts Now! Groom Yourself for Greatness	55
Chapter Four	The Truth about Daddies	69
Chapter Five	A Little Cash Never Hurts!	93
Chapter Six	The Symbiotic Relationship between Child Support and Custody	117
Chapter Seven	Communication with the Baby's Father	143
Chapter Eight	Do I Really Need a Bassinet?	169
Chapter Nine	Your Living Space	181
Chapter Ten	Work/Life Balance	203
Chapter Eleven	Your Baby Shower	223
Chapter Twelve	Birthing Your Way	229
Chapter Thirteen	Into Your Near Future as a Single Mom	243
Epilogue		257
Works Cited		259

Preface

Hello there, and welcome to your new life. Let me tell you a little something about this book you are about to read:

First off, this book is written with the goal of helping single mothers-to-be embrace their destinies as parents and contributing members of society with confidence, competence, and courage. This book welcomes, accepts, and expects readers of all reproductive rights views, spiritual paths, races, ages (with the understanding that most readers will be of child-bearing age), education levels, income levels, and genders (again, with the understanding that the vast majority of readers will be women).

While some readers may not themselves be pregnant, the subject matter of this book will be of the greatest interest to (and will be best understood by) women who are choosing or considering following through with an "unsupported pregnancy." An unsupported pregnancy is a *planned or unplanned* pregnancy in which the child's natural father is absent as the result of his rejection of the mother and/or child, or in which the child's mother has abandoned the relationship with the child's father. Although most of the subject matter in this book can also be appreciated by women in other single pregnancy scenarios (deployment of husband, intentional single pregnancy, widowhood), such readers may find a significant portion of this book's material irrelevant to their experience, but may still benefit from the discussions therein.

This book is meant to cover those issues that are specific to those experiencing unsupported pregnancies with a focus on emotional health, financial health, and work/life logistics. While health issues are addressed and legal issues are discussed at length, specific health issues and particular legal issues within one's state are best discussed with experts in those fields.

This is not a book about "options counseling," the perceived "rights" and "wrongs" of adoption, abortion, or parenting—rather, this is a book specifically for single mothers-to-be. This work honors the free will of its readers and aims to provide unconditional support for its very diverse audience in choosing the path best understood—as well as experienced first-hand—by the author. It is written with the knowledge that a single mother-to-be is every bit as capable of being an excellent parent as any woman who is married or otherwise partnered. The difference in outcomes between these two paths is in the challenges either woman will face and whether or not she is adequately prepared for them.

Finally, this is a book for the reader, not the baby. The comprehensive wellbeing of a child is contingent upon that of its natural mother. A healthy, happy, and empowered parent is a necessary component in the life of a child. In this book, the mother's happiness is the first priority, and the focus on her wellbeing will result in her being a loving, committed, and effective parent.

Introduction

Imagine if you will a typical first grade classroom of twenty-seven children. The children are of various sizes, colors, religions, income levels, and skill levels; their only unifying characteristic being that they are all about six years old. As one who has worked in child care administration, I can attest to the fact that one can assume nothing about a child simply by looking at them. Sometimes the children of the wealthiest parents are dressed in rags and are none too clean. Sometimes the best-behaved child has a stormy home life. Sometimes the blond-haired blue-eyed child is Jewish. Sometimes the little girl whose hair is fixed so perfectly every day is from a low income home. Only after looking in a child's file are their secrets and mysteries revealed: Child #1 lives with his grandparents. Child #2 has a list of fifteen people authorized to pick him up from school. Child #3 is forbidden by his religion to celebrate Halloween. The list goes on. Their circumstances are every bit as diverse as their faces.

Of these 27 children, how many would you guess had been born to single women? Most people seem to think the percentage is rather low, that out of 27 children, only 3, 4, or 5 of them were born to single women. The truth is that roughly one third of those children, nine out of twenty-seven, were born to single women. In 2014, single women set a record with 1.6 million babies. Although many would like single pregnant women to believe otherwise, children from one-parent homes are no longer the extreme minority.

But just as our twenty-seven children vary so greatly in their circumstances, so do their mothers. Of those mothers who were single at the time of their child's birth, several had partners who continued to be active fathers in the children's lives. Some pregnancies were planned, and some were not. Some of those mothers found suitable partners very quickly after their children were born. Some such women take years to find partners, and some never do. One must also consider that some of the mothers who were wed at the time of their child's birth will be divorced by the time the child is in the first grade. A lot can change in six years, after all. Yes, single parent households and blended families are all over the place. Anyone who would have you believe otherwise is not only deceiving you, they're deceiving themselves.

Yet there still seem to be people sold on the idea that single pregnancy and single parenthood is scandalous and unfair to children, casting them into an existence of disadvantage. But this mindset is decreasing in popularity, due to the fact that it's a cultural tenet rather than a logical conclusion—it is belief rather than fact. Doesn't it seem more logical that the child who has one very dedicated parent is much better off than the child whose parents are constantly fighting, in and out of jail, neglectful, or undependable?

Everyone who has grown up on what many would call the "right side of the tracks" has seen examples of children who have every material distraction known to mankind at their fingertips, but no interaction, supervision, or guidance at all, not to mention the absolute nightmares that have been found to exist within some traditional and privileged households. Compare the life chances of the child who lives in such a household to the child whose mother can only offer healthy food, help with homework, and a walking companion to and from school. Which child is more likely to become a contributing member to society? Opinions differ, but I cast my vote for the child with the parent who cares. When we look at these nine out of twenty-seven children who are born to single women, can we really say that they are at a disadvantage to the other students when we can't see into their lives to weigh the pros and cons of their individual situations?

In my opinion, the number one enemy to a child of a single mother is not the child's mother, but is instead the culture that tries to convince this mother that she is somehow inadequate, incapable, or deficient. When a person or group of people subscribes to this belief and makes it known, they are launching an all-out attack against this mother and her child. They are doing this because they *want* this mother to feel that she is deficient so she won't go forward to challenge the closely held cultural tenets that keep her marginalized with her "impossible" and "unexpected" success in her job, her personal choices, and in raising her child. If they succeed in convincing this mother that she is deficient without a partner, who wins? Certainly not the mother, certainly not the child, and certainly not the society in which we live. Those who gain might include politicians in need of a scapegoat for their irresponsible spending, predatory male suitors, insecure women, and pedophiles. That's not the side I want to be supporting—what about *you?*

I am here to help facilitate a different outcome for single mothers-to-be and their children. Single-since-pregnancy mothers can (and do) have money, homes, careers, educations, and lives that we love all while providing an empowering, loving, and healthy atmosphere for our children to grow and thrive—we just have to ignore our detractors, clear away the obstacles, and grab hold of our destinies.

Those who believe otherwise had just better get used to being wrong.

Chapter One

This Was My Wake-up Call

I was twenty-eight years old when I found myself at the most important crossroads of my life: I found that I was the hostess of an unexpected pregnancy.

I had been living an extremely satisfying life thus far: I had graduated from college years before, had taken a year to teach English in Europe, and had since settled into an exciting and comfortable career as a tour guide. I'd had a few loves pass through my life, some of them going on down the road at their insistence and some at mine. I had seen both the good and bad aspects of being in a relationship, and decided that I was better suited for the drawbacks of single life than the drawbacks of being with the wrong person. I did consider that we women have a biological window of opportunity to embrace pregnancy, and that when that window closes, it closes forever.

The relationship that resulted in my pregnancy was so new that I didn't know whether my unborn child's father was this thing they call "marriage material" or not, and I realized that there was a significant chance that he would not want anything to do with me or the child. Despite both of us having been raised Catholic, *I* supported a woman's right to terminate a pregnancy, a viewpoint not shared by my child's father. However, I didn't feel that my personal situation called for any such action. After all, to continue the pregnancy was my first and solid choice. I did not perceive my situation as being a risk to my physical or social livelihood. I had willingly entered into a physical relationship with my child's father knowing the potential consequence of pregnancy. I wanted children someday, why not now? As a bonus, I had a good job, great credit, and a supportive family. I knew it wasn't going to be easy, but I couldn't clearly see where the hard part was going to come in. I was shaken, and I knew life was changing profoundly, but I didn't give other options so much as a passing glance. Barring my own death or a miscarriage, I was going to be a mother.

I told my son's father about my situation in the least invasive way I could. I wrote him a letter excusing him from any involvement if he wished not to be a part of it, but believing that he would want to be involved in our child's life on some level. The only thing I requested from him was his medical history, so I could know what to expect in the way of my child's health. He called when he received my letter, and told me that a medical history was on its way. That's the last I heard from him until long after our son was born. The medical history never came.

Okay, well—I knew where I stood. I was going to have a child very much on my own. Sure, I could sit around for the rest of my life waiting for true love or "the perfect time," but I had seen too many of my friends wait too long for a love or a perfect time that never came. Just because this gift of parenthood had come unexpectedly and without all the traditional hardware didn't mean that I wanted to return it. I also felt as though this challenge were somehow divinely charged, as though God/Creator/Source energy had said, "This gift comes with a lot of responsibility and strength of will. Let's see how you handle it."

Let's just say I had no idea what I had signed up for. I had always been a winner, and had achieved everything in life I had set my sights on. My adult years up until that time had been spent studying literature, learning languages, playing music, shopping for fun clothes, traveling the world, and roaming the forests. I was well aware of the social injustices that happened in far-off lands and at far-off times, but no such injustices could ever touch me, or so I thought. My biggest misconception about my situation was that my choice would be largely respected, and that our society provided easy access to resources and people who were going to help me avoid having an abortion that I didn't plan to have.

It didn't take long for me to see that this was going to be much harder than I thought. Morning sickness had dealt a quick blow to my occupation and income, and my Ob-Gyn bills quickly drained my savings. My friends didn't know what to say or do—this was too heavy for the handful friends that I had made or reconnected with since I moved back home just a year before. Within a few short weeks I found myself living back at my parents' house at the age of 28, wondering what had happened to my perfect life. I found myself in need of some kind of help to get through this—and so my search began.

The first place I looked for help was through various pregnancy counseling services. Sadly, it soon became apparent that their primary concern was that I didn't plan to abort, and their secondary concern was that I find "the right kind of family" to give my child to. They didn't give me any information on custody or child support, financial assistance, legal issues, or support groups. When I didn't fit the expected profile of young, poor, terrified, ashamed, and malleable, they basically threw me out. Some of them seemed to relish the challenge of hurting my confidence in the process: Whatever happened to me or my child after my first fifteen weeks of pregnancy was entirely my problem, and it should be understood by me that the only way to right my wrongs was to give my child to a "real" family, one with a wife and husband (or at least a coupled woman and man) demonstrating "appropriate" gender roles. After all, I had sinned! I was a terrible example of what a woman should be. And any hardship I encountered from this point forward, be it social alienation, financial struggles, or physical ailments, was my penance for having dared copulate outside the sanctity of marriage, or at least a partnership that had been agreed upon with honesty from both parties (I have since grown to understand that the natural father's *approval* of the situation is of great social value). This act of copulation outside a mutually agreed-upon family plan made me *detestable* in the eyes of God, and my example would certainly pervert the destiny of the innocent child who was dealt the misfortune of having to bear the cross of my misdeeds! Wow, thanks for nothing!

And what of the other reproductive rights camp? Might I find some support there? I found considerably less judgment, and for that I am appreciative. However, a movement that dedicates the bulk of its effort to preventing pregnancies and preserving the legality of abortion does not specialize in helping women like me. Furthermore, there seemed to be a prevailing attitude that my choice to continue a pregnancy was a foolish one—not for moral reasons, but for reasons of the social and economic well-being of myself and my country, and it was assumed that what stood between me and making the "right decision" was my lack of education coupled with adherence to an unreasonable fear of a medical procedure that I had been convinced was murder. The message seemed to be, "You don't have to do this, you know. Life will be much better if you don't. If you want to terminate, we can help you. If you don't, you're on your own."

Furthermore, I began to perceive that many players on both sides of the fence, as much as they would hate to admit this, united in a "secret handshake:" Between the choices of parenting and adoption, adoption was considered preferable by both sides. Regarding the choice of parenthood, the literature from the "life" camp would typically throw in a foreboding paragraph or two about how it would be hard to get a man to love me, and how I might miss my prom or other events that my friends were partaking in (logically assuming that only teens find themselves single, pregnant, and looking for help). The "choice" camp gave me nothing at all. It was a bit more honest in that they didn't pretend to specialize in my circumstances.

And what about books and magazines? Could I find any real help there? Despite the predominantly superficial focus of the various pregnancy books and magazines I read, the biggest challenge to my success in this undertaking was *not* morning sickness, stretch marks, weight gain, looking good in maternity clothes, learning the harmful effects of alcohol on a growing fetus, adhering to my birth plan, the price of baby clothes, or anticipation of potential complications during labor and delivery. Instead, the biggest challenge to my happiness and success came directly from those whose ostensible mission was to help me—and the vast majority of these so-called "helpers" just wanted me to follow instructions, as though my quest for help were an admission of my deficiency.

Books and magazines targeted towards a pregnant audience seemed to completely ignore people like me.

Yes, I was alone in this. With all the talk about reproductive rights in our country, it became apparent that the right to peacefully continue a pregnancy as a single woman had been swept under the rug as too confusing a choice to garner any true organized and competent support. I had to be my own best friend, and my help had to come from within.

Many years later, having raised a beautiful, smart, ethical, competent, loving, wonderful son of whom I am extremely proud, and knowing countless other single-while-pregnant women whose children and accomplishments illustrate various successes and dreams come true, the condemnation I experienced seems very far away—like a joke you knew was funny, but you can't remember the punchline. But I remember the pain. I remember wondering during my darker times if I had made a terrible mistake—that they were right: I would live a life of poverty and loneliness with my clothes in tatters and dirty hair, that I'd somehow get addicted to crack, that my son would turn out to be a criminal, and that I had foolishly thrown away my perfect life.

Before I was well past any such fears, I wondered how they could possibly have thought they were doing something productive by playing this destructive and manipulative game of helpful-information keep-away. What I have since learned, and what any single pregnant woman who does not plan to abort should know, is that a healthy baby is a prized commodity—that there are scores of people in this country who would go completely broke to have your baby, and many more people who sit to make a pretty penny off the arrangement (not the mothers of course—it is unethical for a mother to sell her own baby, but it's perfectly fine for someone else to sell it). These stories about how miserable your life will be are just that: stories—fictitious stories. And although you may feel like the only one in the world who is going through this, and may even be suffering social or financial losses as a result of your choice to have a baby, by the time your child is in kindergarten, about a third of your child's classmates will be children of single parents as the result of divorce. Some of those parents will have problems that you will have learned to avoid.

Now we can't blame or judge people for simply wanting babies, but wherever there is a demand for something, there are people hoping to capitalize on that demand by any means possible. So, when people in the pregnancy "help" field discourage you from keeping your baby, are they doing it for money? Whether it's to earn money through an adoption or the belief that they will somehow save money through taxes they don't want to pay, the answer is yes—they are doing it for money.

Now I've got news for everyone who piled their negative projections on me—it's the same news I've got for every single mother-to-be who will listen: Besides a couple of years that I was fumbling through my pregnancy and early motherhood making terrible mistakes one after the other, my life is still pretty darned perfect. And I could run over my list of all the things I have accomplished since my pregnancy, but what's the point of that? My list is not your list. You're a different person—it might not inspire you at all. And the saddest news of all for those people who helped darken those early years, as well as everyone who hopes to gain by the same methods, is that they will have one less victim for every person who reads this book.

And as long as so many people are hung up on the "right thing to do," we might as well examine what that means. If you are one of those people who feels one hundred percent supported in your pregnancy and nobody has tried to moralize with you over your situation, you're one of the lucky ones, and a lot of what is said here will just reinforce what you already know. The rest of you need to ask yourselves these questions in order to become and remain strong:

When you are single and pregnant, what is right, and what is wrong? I will answer that question with another question: What kind of a fool thinks they have the answer to that? Anyone who has paid an ounce of attention has seen how our society has a way of putting single pregnant women in a no-win situation, making them feel as though they, as individuals, are solely responsible for becoming pregnant in the first place—although I have yet to hear of a human woman who successfully fertilized herself without a product that comes from a willing or somehow participating male human (yes, I realize there are exceptions, but I am going to go out on a limb here and assume you did not rape a man).

Most logical people can see that it's impossible for any one person to take on all the conflicting views surrounding sex, birth control, ethics, health, parenting, marriage, and morality, and come up with a "truth" that works for everybody. Take two Christians for example: Jimmy Carter and Sarah Palin. The only similarity is that they both ran for office.

Sometimes it is hard for us to understand exactly what rule we have broken in order to earn condemnation. I myself learned that to follow the rules of Catholicism certainly doesn't earn you any points with Catholics, failing to "burden" the system by not using public assistance doesn't spare you from people believing that you are somehow costing them money, and making your child your first priority in every aspect of your life doesn't shield you from the judgment of people who think that having a child without a father is just plain wrong. So why try to please people like this? If they're determined to dislike you, they will. At the end of the day, you've only got yourself. Do what you need to do to keep yourself financially and emotionally healthy, and don't be ashamed. Be a self that you admire.

Next question: Why is it that people in the pregnancy "help" industry feel such a need to deliver warnings and apply their ideas of right and wrong to various options rather than simply providing information that allows the counselee to make her own decisions about her life path? My conclusion: Unhappy people love to derail other people's lives. Don't let them derail yours.

And finally, there's the issue of hypocrisy. Some of the most hurtful and judgmental people do harmful things in the name of "saving babies." This, ladies, is a ruse. Every person who has ever shamed, ostracized, tormented, or judged a single pregnant woman within her legal window of opportunity to terminate—*including* pregnancy counselors, politicians, doctors, religious leaders, family advocates, family members, adoption placement personnel, or even the child's natural father—has made the option of termination more palatable than single motherhood. If they really do believe that abortion is murder, they had better repent hard before judgment day because they took an active part in loading the "murder weapon." Their judgmental attitudes, their refusal to understand the value of social programs, their failure to help, their refusal to educate, their adherence to patriarchy, their mob mentality, and their attachment to the superiority of the traditional family is not preventing abortion—it's creating a bigger demand for it!

Wouldn't it also follow that anyone who has done any of these things to a single pregnant woman when she is beyond her window of opportunity to safely terminate her pregnancy is a *child abuser*? After all, various studies have concluded that feelings of anger, stress, horror, fear, regret, anxiety, rejection, disappointment, guilt, and shame are transferred from the pregnant woman to the baby inside her, and can cause any multitude of problems that may otherwise not have occurred (which is one of the reasons that it is important for you to learn to shield yourself against emotional attacks). Shouldn't we be trying to minimize this trauma to the baby? Why is it that so many judges give *custody* rights to the "natural fathers" who have insisted upon abortion, tormented women for continuing their pregnancies without their approval, refused to pay child support while insisting on the baby's having their last name, and have threatened to "take the baby away" from the mother by exploiting legal connections and using big piles of money (none of which finds its way to prevent this woman's need to apply for public assistance or to help pay labor and delivery costs)? Could it be that these types of people, and any others involved in this systematic abuse of a pregnant woman are simply.... *child abuse ADVOCATES*?

That said, let's do ourselves a favor and not worry about right or wrong. Whatever you decide to do, however you decide to address your pregnancy, please do not make any decisions under pressure from hypocrites. It is time to recognize them for what they are, and *stand in your power*. And as you will learn—if you haven't already learned—to stand in your power does not mean publicly calling them out as your enemies and trying to get them to see the error of their ways. People like this are blind to their own reflections and you cannot afford to let that be your problem. Standing in your power means having the strength to ignore them and put your energy towards yourself and the awesome, happy life that awaits you.

If a woman's true desire is to continue her pregnancy and become a mother, rarely does she decide to abort or arrange for adoption if she feels safe, empowered, supported, and loved. Part of loving a person is telling them the truth. The truth is this: Being a new single mother, although potentially challenging, is no tragedy. You just need the right tools for it to go smoothly.

Make no mistake about it: The growth you experience through the next couple of years of your life will be painful at times. For this reason, the decision to be a parent has to be yours and yours alone, and should be based on your desire to have and raise this child, whatever this child turns out to be. Don't believe that your child's father will one day magically fall in love with you for the strength you have demonstrated in having this baby, because although it *could* happen, it's really not likely. Don't do it for your family, your friends, or your community. Some of your most enthusiastic supporters will disappear at the first moment that you need their help. Many people outside your circle of friends and family will have an interest in what you do with your body when you are pregnant, but these people are nowhere when you spend your first sleepless night with an agitated baby. You will become acutely aware of every subtle way the various media objectify women, valuing their short-lived sexual appeal and then casting them aside, and you might be angry because this happened to you. Certain television programs, magazines, and popular songs you used to enjoy might make you think harder about what is being said and shown, and you will no longer enjoy them. You will know first-hand that ignorance is bliss, and you may find yourself suddenly and uncomfortably awake and aware—but just like a chiropractic adjustment, the pain goes away when we shift. If this is your first child, the adjustments you make will be many. An idealistic perception of many of your fellow human beings may be the first thing you shed in order to don your new thicker skin.

At this time you might be wondering: If I am an advocate for single pregnant women who want to have their children, why would I be pointing out all the bad things that may not happen? My philosophy is simple: Know your enemy. Only after you've studied the disease can you create its vaccine. And let me tell you, I had a bad case of single pregnancy unreality syndrome, which makes me a good candidate to make sure this vaccine covers all the bases. I got just about every symptom: Despite my years of devotion, I couldn't find any help from my church, and my son's father and his socially prominent religious family refused to even remotely treat me like an honest human being. Pregnancy "counselors" did their best to manipulate me into giving my child up for adoption, relentlessly reiterating that to keep my child would be "selfish" and "harmful." Certain women in my community treated me with fear and mistrust, and certain men in my community joked about me. I didn't get Medicaid because I had too much money in my saving's account and had to pay cash for my labor and delivery (a rule that has since been changed, thank God), yet I was often made aware that I was regarded as a "financial drain on society." My Ob-Gyn treated me as though I had no right to ask for an extra packet of ketchup with my extra-large order of fries. Friends abandoned me, attorneys exploited me, and it seemed that society had thrown me away. Terms like "murderer," "morality," "child abuser," "selfish," and "wrong" were thrown about all willy-nilly until they held no meaning for me whatsoever. I was a kind person. I was a responsible person. Why did people suddenly treat me like I was some sort of disgusting stain?

Thankfully, not everyone suffers to the extent that I did. There's a possibility that you may not! As for the rest of you, I don't want to write your story for you, but I think that reading this book will help ensure that you will be able to see any criticism as an unfortunate waste of someone else's energy, and any challenge to your success and happiness as the temporary condition that it truly is. You might learn quickly that if people leave you, you will find new and better people. If things change, they will be making way for the new.

And despite my hardships, I actually feel privileged that I got to experience these challenges, a sentiment shared by the other mothers who donate their time to our online support group, some of whom had even bigger problems that included domestic violence, familial rejection, wrongful termination, and homelessness with an infant. After all, we can use our collective experience to minimize the likelihood that you will experience these things. Together, we can help women in unsupported pregnancies to make wise, grounded decisions about their futures, to minimize the effects of those forces working against them, and to help them lead the best possible lives. This goal cannot be attained through dishonesty, manipulation, or condemnation. It can only be attained through experience combined with taking an honest, active role in helping others whose circumstances you understand.

And guess what—you can and probably will achieve all that you aim for in life, whether that includes a basic or higher education, home ownership, fitness, a happy marriage, financial stability, or any other measure of success you may have been told is impossible for a single mother to achieve. I myself have knocked most of these things off this list, which at times made me want to gloat to those who had tried to dim me with projections of failure, or laud these things as proof of my worth. But really, it doesn't matter whether you end up rich, married, or highly educated, if that's not how your life plays out, or if you simply change your mind about what you put your energy towards. I consider my greatest achievements to be the triumphs of my spirit: My contentedness that can only come from self-love, and how that contentedness has helped me to raise a happy, ethical, respectful, responsible, and loving person: my beautiful son. I cannot take credit for everything this magnificent soul has decided to be, but I do take credit for creating and enforcing a safe place for him to learn, grow, and be his exceptional self.

Another component of my happiness is to see other women who were at times beaten down and confused, rejected, frightened, abandoned, and harassed transformed into people who are living their dreams, posting happy photos of themselves and their children on Facebook; hearing about their successes, watching them land their dream jobs, seeing them win on Wheel of Fortune, and whatever else gives them joy. Joy is not a finite commodity. The more you share it, the more it grows.

I want the same for you. You are the foundation upon which your child will stand. Let's build you up strong so that nothing can knock you down.

Chapter Two

Banishing the Negative, Cherishing the Positive

Let me start this chapter by saying that I hope you are the happiest person on Earth. I hope you are so secure and so evolved that you can just let everything negative roll off your back, that you don't blame yourself (or anyone else) for any unfortunate thing that happens to you, and that you regard every day of your life as a beautiful gift. However, I expect that you are indeed human like the rest of us, and are subject to some challenges to your mood and disposition as a result.

This chapter will be helpful in a painful sort of way. It will be like ripping the old, stained, damaged wallpaper from the walls, exposing the glue and the awful, icky colors of yesteryear so that you can paint them the new, fresh, vibrant color of your choice. Just like the outdated wallpaper and the icky underneath, we have to address it in order to do anything about it: The tearing down will not be easy, but putting on the fresh paint will be fun. Let's not waste any time. Let's get to remodeling!

Dirt Sandwich Surprise
Upon first becoming a single pregnant woman, I was surprised at the negative treatment I got from both men and women in my community. I didn't think my choice to become a single mother was anyone's business, nor did I think it would be considered a particularly bad choice in any modern adult's opinion—after all, I thought the topic that got under everyone's skin was not single parenting, but abortion. I wasn't having an abortion (not that it would be anyone's business if I were), so what did anyone care what I was about to do?

What I didn't realize was that I was stepping out of the place that our society had reserved for me, and in so doing, not only was I going against the authority of the "ruling" gender, but also those members of the "subordinate" gender who felt that happy parenthood was an indication of status meant to be enjoyed only by those who had followed our culture's rules.

The rules of which I speak are restrictive, widespread, and are accepted by the majority, and there is a complex system put in place to help insure that we women do not dare set one foot out of our place, which is exactly what some people believe you've done by choosing to have a baby despite the absence of your baby's father. Some people will take measures to assure that one foot is as far as you'll go, but do not let them succeed! This pregnancy is not your "punishment" for failing to follow the rules—it is the natural consequence of sexual intercourse that sometimes can't even be prevented with birth control. In the event that in your heart you do feel that your pregnancy is the result of a huge moral mistake, you must forgive yourself and move forward, as it's nobody's job to remind you of your mistakes again and again—and yes, guilt and shame *hurts* you. You will have to polish your spiritual and mental armor to deal with these attitudes in the next two or three years, but in order to truly take control of the situation, you must first understand exactly what's going on.

Rules? What Rules? I Haven't Broken Any Rules!

According to sociologists, our culture has what is called a Social Stratification System, a way of categorizing the status of a person in our society. Throughout our country's history, the people at the top of our social stratification system (the ones in power) have been the white males. If you are non-white or female, no matter how much money, beauty, or strength you have, you are not at the top of our society's food chain. Before you lose any hope, I will assure you that there is a way to step outside of this food chain and protect yourself from getting eaten—and you don't have to turn against your gender, your heritage, or your individual likes and dislikes in order to do it. But in order to do this, you must first see that this food chain does indeed exist.

From the time we are born, we women are conditioned by our culture to be more passive, demure, delicate, and quiet than your average male, even if it is not in our nature to be so. Even if our parents encourage us to hunt, fish, and play ice hockey, we eventually experience pressure (in the form of teasing, ostracism, harassment, missing out on traditional events like the prom, or being passed over for certain jobs) to be what a woman is "supposed to be" according to our culture's standards. To be sure, there is a similar pressure put on the men in our culture: Men are not supposed to cry, to be too pretty, to be soft, to be too sensitive, etc. This too is damaging, but the pressure society puts on us women, particularly mothers, is much more consistent—so much so that sometimes it takes a person pointing it out before we realize that we have been submitting to someone else's idea of what we are supposed to be.

Throughout history, our traditional role as women has been to take care of the children and the house, while the men have been expected to be the providers, to be the public representatives for the family, and to take advantage of the freedom this public life offers. I, for one, would love to cook, clean, and hang out with children all day long, but in doing that, I would be serving my own agenda, and somebody would have to be bankrolling me. It just so happens that I need to bankroll myself, and that's where the situation gets tricky.

Boys and girls in our society are conditioned to embrace these roles from an early age: boys are encouraged to be aggressive, strong-willed, and even violent, whereas girls are taught to be nurturing, passive, to care about their appearance, and to excuse those males for simply doing what they have been taught to do.

As you may very well know by now, we women typically earn 25 percent less in the workplace than men do. There are many sociological reasons for this, but here are two bits of information that might put it into perspective:

1. Our society expects that every woman has a man taking care of her. If she doesn't, our society at large tends to feel that the woman is deficient because she is not minding her traditional place. Many feel that this woman does not deserve to be making as much money as a man. If it does occur to them that some women have to be both the breadwinner and the homemaker of their households, then it's often believed that these women simply aren't good enough women to have been claimed by honest men.
2. Women are often passed up for promotions at work because the behavior we are taught by our culture has undermined our ability to command respect: We apologize for things that are not our fault, we don't make our wants and needs known, and we are silent about our accomplishments. We are also undervalued, as many regard men as the bigger contributors in the workplace.

Although the "man as worker/ woman as homemaker" system may work for some couples, it's putting us modern working mothers in a no-win situation. We're at the bottom of the pay scale and often have to pay for childcare. Of the time we have left, most of it goes towards caring for our children, not ourselves.

If you have decided to continue with an "unsupported" pregnancy (a pregnancy without the approval or participation of your child's father), you have stepped outside the traditional role of what our culture thinks you're supposed to be. In some people's opinions, you need to be taught a lesson: You need to mind your place. The "place" that we are to "mind" is beneath that of men and coupled women. In our society, we women are taught to respect a man's "authority," or his right to tell us what to do.

When you are attuned to this, you see it all over the place. Take for example a friend who wants to buy a piece of furniture you have decided to get rid of. She and her husband are both teachers, so they are equal financial contributors to the household. She has expressed interest in this piece of furniture throughout the years. You offer her a more than fair price—and it's less than one hundred dollars, so it's less than your friend takes home for one day of work. Then she says she has to ask her husband. Days later, she sends you a message. She tried. The answer is no.

Until rather recently, women were regarded as property. A wife was part of the master's estate. Sure, some women in history were loved and cherished, but for a woman to step out of her traditional role usually caused her husband social shame, which sometimes compromised his ability to make a living and to keep respect amongst his peers (which was central to making a living). A woman had a duty to her husband and her family to mind her "gender role" manners. If a woman didn't do what her husband wanted, he could beat her. After all, she was really no different than an ox who refused to pull a cart.

Some of you might be backpedaling right now. *"But I was willing to follow the rules. I would have been happy in a traditional relationship. I was a perfect girlfriend. He said he was going to marry me. The father of my baby deceived **me**."* Although you have all *my* understanding and all *my* sympathy, in the opinion of the majority of our population, you're not the important one—*he* is. And according to our culture's rules, he's allowed and is even encouraged to have premarital or extramarital sex—you're not.

This is one reason why sexually open women are often referred to as "trash." They don't fit the description of what traditional men want in a wife. As a result, they are perceived as having no importance, and society throws them away by refusing to take care of them. After all, a woman who can't be controlled is too much of a liability for a busy rule-abiding man to take care of.

You may have noticed that there is a social stratification system even within the community of single pregnant women. Within our community, there are several sub-groups, but there are two such groups that I will mention for the sake of your understanding our culture's unspoken subordination agreement with men.

Group 1: Married and abandoned

Some single mothers are eager to distinguish themselves as having been married to their child's father at the time of their child's conception. These women are in every bit as much of a bind as the rest of us are, but many of them feel the pressure to make sure that everybody knows that their husbands were present and willing to be parents at the time of conception. In some cases, the marriage may have fallen apart as a result of marital misbehavior on the part of this very woman, but the marriage saves her from having to bear public speculation on her marital conduct.

Long after my pregnancy, I came into contact with one such woman. After mentioning the similarities in our situations, she wanted to make sure that I understood those similarities to be only in my imagination, her point punctuated with a shaking finger: "No,

I was *married* when I became pregnant. There is a big difference between what I did, and what *you* did."

Before I go on, it should be known that *most* married and abandoned pregnant women I have come into contact with have not had this attitude. Most of them will be the first to raise their hands and proclaim, "We're just the same, you and me!" But the fact is that they are not often safe to do so because judgment is everywhere. To be perceived as "loose" in some communities can result in a dangerous social climate for a woman and her children. Sometimes a woman will do what she feels she must do in order to survive, and sometimes that includes distinguishing herself from people who may be perceived as low.

Group 2: Unmarried-but-partnered women
In many cases, the unmarried-but-partnered woman gets the best of both worlds: She has outsmarted the system. Not only does she enjoy the benefits of a partnership without the legal confines of a marriage, but she also has the freedom to leave the relationship without losing whatever may have always been hers. Another bonus: If she doesn't work or has a low income, she can often qualify for Medicaid in the event that she doesn't have insurance.

It should be noted that this is a very diverse group of people. Some of them are avoiding marriage because they're not sure their partner is "the one." Some of them really want to be married to their partners, but their partners are balking. Sometimes it is a completely mutual relationship and the two are simply waiting for the right time to marry. Some have no intentions of ever getting married, but want to live as "life partners." Some are just getting what they can get while they can get it. Some would rather not strike out on their own—not everyone can happily do that. Yes, some of them are simply codependent, don't have a long-term interest in their partners, and will upgrade as soon as they find someone more pleasing.

Regardless, these women tend to forget that they are still in fact single. Why? Because our society forgets. After all, if there is a man present and willing to authorize and supervise the situation, then no major crime against our culture has been committed.

Both the above examples demonstrate our culture's tenet that what a woman does is all okay, so long as there's a man who approves of (and will oversee) the situation. If we adhere tightly to this belief, then it would seem that single pregnancy without a man's approval is *more wrong* in that there is a man whose autonomy has been sacrificed for the choices made outside his validation. Many people feel that a man who has contributed to an unwanted pregnancy has been made a victim: his reputation, his paycheck, and even his sperm have been held hostage for the sake of some "insignificant" woman's wild agenda. If this man admits and honors his responsibility, then the shame that normally accompanies a woman's single pregnancy is excused. If he doesn't, then many believe that the woman is to blame.

Is this fair? Is this right? Is this what God wants? The answer is no. This is simply the result of individuals neglecting to question the rules of our culture and allowing a patriarchal society (a society that honors men above women) to flourish.

Friends, it is time to be aware. When you are aware of the forces that are working against you, you can begin to make change.

Luckily for you, what our culture thinks you should be is not necessarily what you are. You are a human being with every right to participate in any human activity, to exhibit any characteristic, and subscribe to any standard that you want. The sooner you realize that you have these rights, the more you will be freed from the enslavement of a society that puts men before women. Furthermore, there are many career paths that even out the playing field: Commission-based sales, cosmetology and hair design, law, and medicine are a few careers in which a person's income will be determined by their effort and talent, as opposed to being deemed worthy by someone of authority.

People in our culture seem to eschew the word "feminism." I personally am not into labels, and this is one that has so many subcategories that it is impossible to come up with a definition that works for everyone. But what I hope to demonstrate is this: You don't have to label yourself in order to recognize that patriarchy is real, and it will likely be the source of any frustration you encounter during your pregnancy and single parenthood.

I personally have no problem calling myself a feminist, but I realize that when I do, people may either get the wrong idea about me, or be extremely confused—and I will not ask that you do the same. I wear dresses more often than pants, I love high heels, I wear makeup, I belly dance, I love fashion, I enjoy cooking and housekeeping, and I like to make myself (by my own definition) pretty. I have no interest in climbing the highest mountain or killing any animals unless I somehow needed to do so. But at those times in my life that I was doing what is traditionally a man's job (driving tour buses) and finding out during casual conversation that I was making four dollars an hour less than my male coworkers—many of whom had wives who packed their daily lunches and were living mostly on their retirement from the jobs they'd had when they were my age—it got to me. Even these co-workers were surprised and incensed to learn my hourly wage. When I was working in human resources for an oil company and could see that the 55-year-old woman who had been competently doing her job for fifteen years made less than the newly-hired twenty-something male in the same position, I paid attention. Patriarchy is something we need to be aware of in order to mitigate. If a man who takes me out does not quickly pick up the check, he will get no second date—and will pay anyway.

That said, the feminist movement in its various forms and stages is your friend. Some of the popular concerns may not resonate with you, but others will.

The Joy of Breaking Restrictive Rules

If your independent spirit has transformed you into the kind of woman that the average man will not be interested in, that is something to celebrate. Why? Because you do not want to date the average man—you want to date only the evolved man, the one who sees you and your child as human beings.

Believe it or not, this is actually cause for celebration: "average" men are those that a smart and empowered woman should never in a million years be interested in, so be thankful that they are automatically eliminated from your radar. Now you are the kind of woman whom the intellectually and morally evolved minority will respect and cherish! You have stepped outside your subordinate position and have made a decision, despite society's rules and expectations, to act on what you feel in your heart is right for you, and you haven't let anyone hold you back. You are going to be a wonderful mother, and if you get married, you will be loved for the strong and independent person you are.

As long as you've become so good at breaking rules, here are a few more that you can break, and be a better person—and a better parent—for it.

#1. Teach your children to respect women.

One of the main reasons people in our society adhere to gender roles is because we've been taught gender roles from the time we are born. Children see men giving women orders all the time, and they see women following these orders. In your household, you must have authority over yourself and be a good example to your children about how a person should be treated. In the event that you include a man in your life, make sure he treats you with respect, and make sure he knows that his presence does not give him the authority to override your standards.

As a single mother, you must behave in a way that defies negative stereotypes of women. You must trust your inner voice and make your own decisions. You can be sensitive without being frail and weak-minded. You can be tender without being a pushover. There will be times when you have to stand up for yourself and be forceful—don't worry about how others perceive you if you step outside the confining role that society has built for you. Your children are developing the habits and ideas that will follow them throughout their lives. Show them the way to be.

When you hear your children say things like "Only boys can play hockey," gently correct them by reminding them that although most hockey players are indeed men, all people have a right to take part in any activity they choose. When your children say that "Only girls play with dolls," remind them that actions figures are dolls too, and that any child who denies himself an enjoyable activity is missing out on one of the pleasures of life. When children learn to perceive themselves and others as human beings with rights to do whatever they please, the battle between the sexes will start to go into remission.

#2. Treat your children like human beings no matter their gender.
If your son does not like to play sports, respect his individuality and foster the interests that he does have. If your daughter is interested in martial arts and doesn't seem to care at all about baby dolls or dressing up, applaud her. If your son wants to wear toenail polish, let him. Accept your child for who he or she is right now—your child might change, and might not. How willing do you think your children will be to let you into their lives and homes if they've always felt inadequate, judged, and guided against their personal dreams? If you introduce your children to a variety of activities, they will show you who they are, and as human beings, they have a right to be who they are. If their natural talents and interests are fostered, they are more likely to be successful in their adulthood. If children feel that they were stifled and misguided in their childhood, they might have identity problems that will follow them into adulthood. What good mother wants her children to feel inadequate and place limits on their potential? Accept your children for who they are, and give them the opportunity to shine and prosper!

#3. Let your children know the difference between nudity and sexuality.
In the United States, our prevailing culture is indeed a bit sexually repressed, which has led to their being sexually obsessed. Most people (both women and men) grow to adulthood having only seen nudity in the form of air-brushed, photo shopped bodies in sexually enticing photographs like those in Playboy. As you can understand, many girls grow up hating their bodies, hating their weight, hating their breasts, and thinking that they are somehow deformed because they have body hair. Similarly, many boys grow up believing that women naturally look like the women in soft-core porn magazines, and that nudity is an indicator of sexuality rather than the simple state of being without clothes.

Although it is not practical for many people to hang out in the nude, for children to witness shameless, incidental, non-sexual nudity is actually good for them. If children are basically familiar with human anatomy, their chances of mistaking nudity for sexuality are decreased. When my son would walk in the bathroom while I was in the bath (which will happen when you are the only parent caring for a child), it was no big deal. If ever I were to slip on the floor and knock myself out, I would expect him to react to my being unconscious rather than being shocked and shamed by my nudity. If we were watching a movie with incidental nudity, he didn't react with incredible interest. He is not critical of himself or others because he knows we all have bodies under our clothes.

One year we took a trip to Czech Republic and found many men and women swimming in public, in the creek, without clothes. People were not staring at each other, handling each other, or invading each other's space in any way. Although most Americans would react with shock or embarrassment, for my son it was no big deal—time to go swimming, trunks or no trunks.

When I lived in Spain, I was pleasantly surprised at the level of comfort that most people had with their bodies. Because it is a very warm country, it is practical that people feel they have a right to shed their clothes in certain situations, and it is understood that just because a person is not dressed, that does not mean that they are offering their bodies for sex. Even my teen-aged male students were horrified at the thought that some American men successfully used the fact that a woman was scantily clad as an excuse to violate her. Such a mindset is extremely suspect in a culture that is not overly sensitive to nudity. It should be every bit as suspect in ours, but we've got a long way to go.

#4. Allow your kids to love all races—they'll have more friends that way

Just like the fact that we are all naked under our clothes, we are all human beneath our skin. All children should be proud of their ethnicity, their heritage, and their uniqueness, but skin color is a physical feature, period. Although persons of various ethnicities and cultures will behave in ways that may be foreign to us, and some have been (and are still being) oppressed by individuals, groups, and the prevailing culture; behavior differences and cultural differences are not natural—they are learned. If children are not made aware of the perceived differences in our value as human beings, they will not perpetuate them.

Children are closer to the divine in that their transition from spirit into a physical form occurred rather recently, which might be why it is harder for children to understand racial "differences." Children seem to be able to understand that a person is more than just a body. Wouldn't it be nice if everyone could tap into that great source of wisdom that is so close to our children?

Yes, in our physical world we are blessed with diversity. Children seem to know that physical differences don't have any bearing on an individual's value. We should open our minds and learn from our children, and mirror that wisdom back to them by teaching children to have pride in their culture, heritage, and ethnicity without categorizing them. Although children will eventually learn the history behind racial inequality in our culture, a child's fundamental perceptions of racial differences (or lack thereof) are taught in the home. If our children are taught to honor all people as human beings, they will have a greater chance of getting along with everyone, and will have a better chance at social, spiritual, and financial success as adults.

#5. *Trust Your Intuition & Teach Your Children to do so As Well*

We have been taught by our culture that reality is defined by what we can perceive through our eyes, ears, or skin, and that something isn't real unless it is manifest in material form. We are taught to *ignore* our feelings, when in reality, our feelings are the realest things we have, especially those that cannot be explained. We are told that to make decisions before we know all the facts about a person or situation is "stupid." Sometimes our reactions to people or situations can be so strong that we develop anxiety, or that we feel a sour or dark feeling that we fight hard to get through, telling ourselves that this doesn't make sense.

Many other cultures, however, know that our intuition is an inner guiding system, and that it is there to help us when the material evidence necessary to make a safe decision is lacking. In some belief systems, one's intuition is regarded as the voice of the Holy Spirit that dwells within us, or the promptings of a guardian angel. Anyone familiar with the chakra system knows that the 6th chakra, also commonly known as the Indigo Chakra or the Third Eye, can be of great assistance to us when it is healthy, and that its health might be compromised when our families tell us that we didn't see something that we did see (imagine catching dad smoking when he promised your mother that he had quit and being told you didn't see anything), when our spiritual side is disregarded (friends mocking you after you told them you had a dream about buildings falling the night before 9/11), or when we fail too many times to heed its warnings.

Most parents will refrain from taking an action that will harm the health of their children. Make a promise that you are going to foster good intuitive health in your child, and that you are going to offer yourself the same consideration. Let your children share the truth that they see. Let them believe that their dreams do mean something. When they tell you things that are fantastic, don't treat it as though they are telling you a lie. If your child sees something confusing that needs to be explained, sit down and explain it to them. If you are at a loss for an explanation, simply be open to their wisdom.

Furthermore, when you are a parent, it is absolutely imperative that you listen to your own intuition about people, places, situations, and anything else that can affect you or your child. Sometimes it is possible to investigate these conflicted feelings you have about something or someone while keeping your child at a safe distance, but if you cannot keep your child at away from someone or something that makes you nervous, eliminate it from your life. You can *always* find another boyfriend. You can *always* find another baseball coach. You can *always* find another apartment, church, or group of friends. It's much better to never know why something felt wrong than it is to learn the hard way that you were right all along.

Even if someone who gives you the intuitive itch is referred and vouched for by a trusted friend, make your own decisions about this person. Just because you trust this friend's opinion, or feel that she must know more than you because she is incredibly financially or emotionally successful in her own life, this doesn't mean that you should turn your back on your own inner guiding system—after all, you have a different life, life circumstances, and life path than this friend of yours. It might be more imperative that *you* stay away from the person in question, which is why her intuition didn't flare up and yours did.

We need to do right by our children, and give them better than what we were given. We need to teach them to live freely, love freely, and honor the spirits that dwell within them. We don't do anything positive for them when we teach them to judge, condemn, or limit themselves or others. Our generation (and others before us) has had to follow some ridiculous rules of conduct put in place by a misguided culture, and it has only served to twist our potential and distort our self-concept. Let's give our children the tools to achieve wisdom beyond what we have experienced. Let's put love and self-respect in the middle of our culture, and watch our children's standards develop beautifully around the powers of goodness, acceptance, and kindness.

Some People Say the Dumbest Things
Imagine you are browsing through the baby department at your local department store. You're getting an idea of what's available, making an imaginary list of what you'll include on your registry for your baby shower, familiarizing yourself with things you never knew existed, and you're having an all-around positive experience and a good day.

Down the aisle you see Jane, a friendly acquaintance from high school. She was always nice to you, and you had good times together working on your high school newspaper. You've heard through the grapevine that she's married and has two kids. Maybe she's got some sound advice for you. Maybe she'll be happy for you. You decide to flag her down and say "hi."

"So, what's new in your life?" She asks.

"I'm having a baby," you answer. "I'm due in March."

"Are you married?" She asks.

"No."

"Who's the father? Do I know him?"

"You might," you answer, "but he doesn't want to be involved."

"Oh, you poor thing," she answers, rolling her eyes. "If there's anything I've learned from having two of my own, it's that babies *need* fathers."

You feel your positive attitude fading while Jane proceeds to boast about her perfect job, her accomplishments, her new house... Suddenly you're embarrassed. You feel rejected and inadequate. It's not your fault that your baby's father wants nothing to do with you or your baby. All you could do is be yourself and listen to your conscience, and that wasn't enough. You feel that you should have known better than to share your news with your old friend. This is going to be a rotten day after all.

Get ready, ladies, these kinds of things are going to happen again and again before it's all over. Sometimes well-meaning people say insensitive things because they simply haven't considered the complexity of your feelings, but more often than not, people who make negative comments do so because they are dissatisfied with their own lives and want to take the heat off themselves.

Take for example our fictitious Jane, who may have her own ugly can of proverbial worms waiting for her at home. Is Jane really happy in her situation? Maybe not. Maybe Jane's husband does nothing but watch football all day while Jane's at work, and her great job is all she has to hold on to. What if Jane's husband goes out to strip clubs every week and comes home with an empty wallet and lipstick on his collar? It's possible that Jane's kids are more than she can handle and she wishes she had waited longer to have her second child. Maybe Jane is so emotionally unstable that she could never handle your situation. Could it be that Jane's father left home when she was a child, never paid child support, never visited her, and Jane is still dealing with her anger over this? It's also possible that Jane and her husband might be on the brink of defaulting on their mortgage, and their lovely new home might be just a lovely memory in days to come. Maybe Jane is beginning to see that she has done herself a great disservice by following our culture's limiting and oppressive "rules."

Not that you should feel triumph in any of these speculations, but it is possible, even probable, that Jane is not the happy person she pretends to be, and if you know these things to be true, it is spiritually and socially correct of you to be the better person and keep your mouth shut. Happy, spiritually evolved people are always positive, which is what you should strive to be, even in the face of those who it seems are trying to tear you down. Sometimes they are not trying to tear you down, but are instead very miserable, insecure, or desperate themselves. They deserve your pity.

Although I used to be the kind of person who avoids confrontation, single pregnancy has shown me that when someone is consistently negative, you have to call them on it. After all, they truly might not know that their negativity is hurting you. A lot of people subscribe to the idea that they are being good friends by "preparing you for the worst," so you don't go dancing off into la-la land thinking that everything's going to be rosy only to be knocked off your feet by a negative outcome. I have found that most of the time, these people don't understand that you've already examined all of the negative possibilities—that you deal with them every day in the privacy of your own mind! You *know* that things might turn out badly, but what good does it do you to dwell on the bad when you can aim towards the best possible outcome?

The recent negative words of a friend reminded me of one of my son's old video games based on the battle of Stalingrad in World War II: A group of soldiers are on a boat heading to the battle at Stalingrad. Some of the soldiers, overcome with fear, jump from the boat and are shot and killed by the commanding officer. Although it might seem extreme (and no, I am not recommending that you shoot your friends), if those soldiers do not believe that they can win this battle, their pessimism does their mission more harm than good. In a sense, if your friends are unwilling to believe in you and fight alongside you, you must tactfully tell them that their mere presence is too much of a risk to your mission of positive thinking. If the negative outcome that they foresee does indeed come true and they bolster it with an "I told you so," it hurts you. You lose a little bit of faith in yourself, and your "friend" reaps some strange, destructive benefit from withholding her belief in you. You have a right and an obligation to follow your own life path and learn your own lessons in your time. Sometimes mistakes are made, but you learn lessons more completely if you are allowed to learn them your own way.

Unfortunately, despite your efforts to enlighten your acquaintances to their insensitivity, negativity, or prying, they might continue to bring up things that you don't want to talk about and that aren't their business. They might feel that their methods are sometimes productive and therapeutic, but these methods are ineffective, and unless they are paid licensed professionals hired by you (and even then), you don't have to appease them with your cooperation. A good way to deal with them is to tell them that the best thing for you right now is to surround yourself with positive influences because you've made your decision, and if they can't be positive for you, they need to give you some space until they can. You have every right not to discuss the worst of what you're feeling. These feelings should be explored under your terms, not theirs.

And finally, don't be afraid to "let people go." I have had countless "changings of the guards" since my pregnancy, and I feel that a lot of it was because for the first time in a long time, I had to be the strong mother my son deserved, whereas I'd made a habit of appeasement for many years prior out of my own fear of abandonment. Sometimes I endured extremely disrespectful or even abusive treatment because I didn't want to be left without friends and I wasn't confident that I could find new ones. Sometimes when the out-of-balance treatment would continue for too long, the universe would make the difficult decision for me: The substandard friend in question would find a reason not to be my friend anymore, and I would think back on all the years of abuse I took and be doubly angry that they had the nerve to find fault with me after all I had endured. However, after going through a fearful and painful phase of shedding a few of these out-of-balance friendships, I started to experience something extraordinary: Every time someone left my life, someone else with similar likeable qualities would cosmically present themselves as a replacement. One characteristic that was always lacking in this new friend was whatever it was that caused the last friendship to be out of balance, as though God could see and acknowledged both what I had longed for and what I could no longer accept. At one point the flip-over had happened three times in seven months, which was frightening. I was developing detachment for people. I asked myself, "Am I ever going to find the people that are going to stay with me forever?" As well as, "What's the point in having people in my life if they're just going to leave?" But I would also ask myself, "Is it better than it was before?" As well as, "Do I still feel that I was systematically mistreated?" The answer was yes. "Would I accept the refusal of this other person to take responsibility for my mistreatment to have that friendship back?" The answer was no.

At this time, I have learned to accept that some people's roles in one's life are temporary. You may be familiar with the phrase: "People come into our lives for a reason, a season, or a lifetime." If someone is in your life temporarily and either has to leave or is sent away, it doesn't mean that either party is bad, it simply means that every individual has a unique evolutionary path. Sometimes we find someone whose path is similar to ours, or someone who exhibits enough pleasing behavior and loyalty for us to greatly appreciate this person despite our differences. Very occasionally, the friendship lasts until one friend passes on. Sometimes it doesn't. Either way, it's a learning experience that helps us to grow in one way or another.

Part of honoring yourself is to stand up for who you are, how you feel, what you think, and to have no shame in defending yourself. As I've said before and will say again, you've got to be your own best friend. If you allow the negativity of ill-wishers to get you down, you've lost one of the many battles. And although it's always a good idea to be generous and loving towards your friends, make certain that this generosity and love is mirrored back to you, and the water in your heart's well is replenished regularly by your inner circle of friends. Otherwise, your heart might grow bitter and hardened from trying to draw water from an empty well—a heart that's taken abuse for too long doesn't open very easily, and you're going to need a healthy, open heart for the years to come. Let your mind and your soul be the armor against your adversaries, and insist on appropriate treatment from the people in your life. You and your baby deserve this.

Mantras and Meditations: Let the Healing Begin!
Although occasionally there exists a person who is enlightened beyond the tendency to feel anger, the fact is that most of us have a lot of it. After coming to the realization that society aims to keep women powerless while dealing with all that comes with an unexpected pregnancy, you might be understandably furious. Although it is natural for a person to feel fear and anger, you must do your best to keep it under control, as too much anger is going to hurt you and your child, even if it's directed at someone else, and fear only serves to cripple you.

This is not to say that severity is never appropriate. There will be times that you will need to be unswerving and use your austerity without hesitation: Custody battles, protecting your child, standing firm in your boundaries, banishing the presence of a lover who keeps you on an emotional roller coaster... The key to appropriate use of your anger is being able to channel it when it's useful, and banish it when it's not.

Following are a few visualization exercises to help you gain control over negative emotions so you can move through these next few months without being crippled by anger.

For those of you who are experienced in the art of meditation, you may have a more complex process or routine you would like to follow during this visualization exercise. If you are new at this, you can get yourself in the right frame of mind by getting yourself comfortable by entering rhythmic breathing (see below), maybe lighting a candle, lighting some incense, and putting on some soft music that doesn't inspire you to sing along, doesn't make you feel like dancing, and doesn't make you try to figure out the chords on your guitar (nature sounds tapes are recommended for musicians). Close your eyes and concentrate on relaxing every part of your body from head to toe.

There are many effective styles of rhythmic breathing, but in my opinion, the easiest is to take slow and easy inhalations to the count of seven, and then exhale to the count of seven about eight times, and continue this breathing throughout the exercise. Concentrate on filling yourself with bright light from above and below, the earth and sky, and expanding it out into the world around you.

Cutting Cords of Attachment

When you have been in a relationship intimate enough to conceive, there is a chance that you and your child's father have developed what are called etheric cords of attachment. These are like energetic wires that stretch between people who have a certain kind of relationship, allowing souls to stay connected for the thousands of years humans lived on Earth before we had such things as phones and the Internet. Etheric cords are why mothers sometimes know when their children are in trouble, friends call when you need them, or why you know who is calling you before you check the caller ID. While cords are originally formed to telepathically share information between people who are close, they are sometimes left in place after a relationship goes sour, and need to be cut in order to turn off the mental arguments or emotional exchange.

In the event that you can't stop thinking about someone, feel the need to find out what they are doing, find yourself tempted to go back into the (or go into another) toxic relationship, find yourself always processing injustices you suffered at their hands, or have imaginary debates or discussions with them, there is a chance that you have these etheric cords between you. While it is natural and normal for processing the demise of a relationship to continue throughout a resulting pregnancy, most people can tell when the processing has gone too far and affects their ability to live and take positive action in the moment. As is mentioned several times in this book, yes—there is a chance that this relationship will repair or be workable, but it does not do you or anyone else any good to be unable to live between now and then—and this won't compromise those chances. Rather, it may improve them, as the parties involved with have to play fair by acting and communicating rather than ruminating and imagining.

While this process sometimes needs to be repeated several times in order to work, it is important to cut these cords. In my opinion, most of the time that a single mother-to-be makes a decision out of concern for the child's father instead of herself, as (for example) in allowing a man to have access to the child without paying child support or a commitment of consistency, the decision was made because the father's more intimate thoughts and insecurities were transferred through etheric cords. The problem with that is that many people have thoughts that they don't act upon in the real world, so that can't be your problem or your baby's problem. If you are conflicted about any aspect of what you owe to yourself, it could distract you long enough for your enemy to get the upper hand.

This is how it's done: Concentrate on communicating with God, your higher self, Jesus Christ, helpful angels or guides… whatever fits your spiritual belief. Ask them to help you and offer their protection while you cut the cords and send all of the energy they were transmitting back to the original sender. You can use any visualization you choose, whether it's God actually cutting the cords for you, or you simply watching them dissolve, knowing that you are divinely supported in this decision.

Repeat this process whenever you find yourself having an imaginary conversation with your child's father, are feeling guilty about the results of his choices, feeling sorry for him, read over old texts (in **Chapter 7** we will discuss the need to keep them, but not look at them), feel tempted to look at his Facebook page or drive by his house or place of work, or anything that is going to reenergize the connection. You may have to do this several times, and sometimes the connection will be reenergized by one or the other of you. But this is the first step in energetically healing yourself.

Exorcising the Ex
Many single pregnant women go through their pregnancies feeling tainted with the energy of rejection or manipulation from their children's fathers, feelings of inadequacy, and feelings of being a victim. Some people successfully address this energy through various modalities: Qi Gong spiritual renewal, Shamanic Soul Retrieval, and good old fashioned prayer. One of my most effective "energy removals" happened when I had just had enough of being sad, and I yelled out, "God, I am desperate now. I see no reason for feeling this pain any longer. It is not serving my higher purpose, and it is unfair to my child. Remove this pain from me!" Interestingly, the next few days were the first few days

in almost a year that I hadn't thought of the ex whose memory had been plaguing me. Isn't it nice when someone listens?

However, most of the time, crying out to God doesn't work. I feel that is at these times that the Divine wants to see us heal ourselves. Following is a visualization to repeat as many times as necessary to help you cleanse and control your beautiful soul from the negative energies of your ex.

Visualize yourself inside a bubble of light. The atmosphere inside this bubble is clean, bright, iridescent, and beautiful. You are wearing shiny, silky, flowing clothes in colors that make you feel powerful in a heavenly way (mine are bright sky blue and ivory embroidered with threads made of real gold). Your skin and hair are clean and clear. This bubble represents your body and your soul. You are perfectly comfortable here, and everything is soft and welcoming. Nothing can trespass here without your express permission.

But something *has* trespassed here into your world. How did it get in? It got into your bubble when you weren't paying attention or you invited it in when you didn't know any better: it is the essence of someone who did not have your best intentions in mind.

Think about this person. Identify the place in your body where you feel a twinge of something not right. Is it your abdomen? Your heart? Your throat? Wherever it is, imagine that it's a dark spot. Surround it and trap it with the brightest light you can imagine (interestingly, when you do this, sometimes you can feel it move, but keep your grip on it or follow it with your light bubble). One you feel like you have it contained, move it out of your body (sometimes people do this through the mouth, coughing it out, even gagging), push it outside your bubble, and then extend a beam of light to push it far away. Once it is gone, it is outside your world and cannot come back.

Repeat the exercise as many times as you like. Your space is now clean. All the negative energy is gone. You are strong, bright, and ready to embrace your beautiful life. Nothing can invade this bright sanctuary without your permission, but if you let your guard down and something bad gets in, you know how to get it out again.

Now it is time to fill your bubble with all good things: love, joy, enthusiasm... the iridescent border of your bubble is like a movie screen. Use it to project all that you aim for in life. Imagine yourself and your baby in a beautiful environment: A sunny day in a meadow surrounded by wildflowers and butterflies, a glorious day at the beach, the two of you living in the home of your dreams, visiting your relatives... whatever makes you feel good. Even if you think your logical mind won't accept this as reality, make it your reality for those few moments—your future just might surprise you.

Dealing with Social Anxiety

Yes, it happens all the time: Someone you work with, someone you're close to, or someone you don't even know exhibits a violent emotional outburst, and although you are *never* the cause of anyone else's lack of control, you are made to feel as though it's all your doing. At certain times in my life, I lived in fear of the next violent outburst I would find myself party to, as my energy was attracting this scenario again and again.

Once while my son was still an infant, I went to the post office to mail several extremely late thank-you cards to the people who had given me gifts at my baby shower. My son was sleeping in the back seat of my car, so I pulled up to the drive-up mail receptacle to mail my letters. Within moments, a man with an extra-long pickup pulled up behind me, and was impatient with the amount of time it took me to get almost a hundred thank-you cards in the box, as he was planning to exit the parking lot.

"Oh, my God," he said, loud enough to ensure I could hear him. "Jesus f***king Christ."

I continued to stuff the box, but I was getting shaky.

"Lazy bitch! Why can't you just go into the post office like everyone else?"

I had a perfectly legitimate reason: my son was sleeping, and I didn't have a bag to carry my mail in. Besides, this was the drive-up mailbox. Any person with a normal sized car could have gotten around me. And as a CDL driver, I personally could have moved a 28-passenger motor coach around my car in less than forty-five seconds. I started to shake, so much so that I dropped my letters, and thus had to operate in this man's radar for even longer. I could feel the anxiety dripping from my stomach into my hands—I could hardly pick my letters back up.

More insults were pelted by this insecure man before my task was finished. I drove away so shakily that honestly, I shouldn't have been driving at all.

But it's not as though he could have physically hurt me—we were in a parking lot, and people were nearby, but I felt vulnerable. I felt hated and rejected by men—I felt like a "throw-away" person: My son's father shown that he didn't care whether I or my son lived or died, and it seemed as though this man could intuit the fact that I was the wolf who was kicked out of the pack and left to fend for herself after she had been exhausted of her uses.

I desperately longed for my dad to be with me, to show this man that I *was* important after all. He would have said, "Hey, buddy. Maybe if you can't drive that thing, you might consider investing in a car that you can handle." Any further resistance would have earned this guy speculation on which inadequacies he might have been trying to camouflage with such a huge vehicle, or a warning that he didn't calm down he might die of "testosterone poisoning," and we would have laughed at this man's rage as we drove away, antagonistically slowly. But it wouldn't have gotten that far: Nobody messes with a six foot three man.

But that was the "me" of yesterday. The "me" of today would have calmly pointed out that this is the drive-up mailbox, and I might have continued with something like: "Come on now, you got yourself in that position. It's not geometrically impossible to get yourself out. These parking lots are designed so you can go around me. Just back up and pull a little bit wider. You can do it!" I would have reacted calmly and fearlessly, and would not have allowed the situation to escalate.

Any further interaction would have been simply ignored, but it wouldn't have gotten that far. Nobody messes with a five foot five single mother. Know why? I have learned the secret to protecting myself from being manipulated by other people's anger, and I thank God that I learned this skill before too much longer, as it's a skill that every parent needs to have in order to lead a happy life. Part of integrating this skill into your life requires knowledge that if any such person doesn't feel a certain measure of success while insulting or intimidating you, he will not continue to do so.

While it is always important to quickly get yourself out of any situation that is truly unsafe (situations where a person is yelling, is on drugs, has a weapon, or is behaving violently), most of these little pissing contests that people get into in public are just that: pissing contests. The key to shielding yourself from other people's energy is to step outside yourself, detach yourself from the physical world, and realize that this life of yours is a movie and you have chosen to play the starring role. Simply and calmly watch the movie, knowing that you're the star, and the script is designed to make you the hero. The person who is causing the strife is simply an insignificant extra in your movie, and their outburst is just an act. He's not even real. He's simply a reflection of your own insecurity. He can't touch you in any way. Pity him. How horrible it must be to have so much negative energy running through your body. You're not going to let the same thing happen to your precious body over some insignificant, two-dimensional character—your body has to last for many years, and you have to take care of it. Don't laugh or sneer, fire back, or do anything that will encourage the behavior. Instead, just be the confident, mature woman who responds calmly… or ignores it completely.

Mantra for Embracing Your Future
Enter into rhythmic breathing and close your eyes, concentrating on drawing energy in from the top of your head and the base of your spine, and from the center of the earth back up to your heart. Feel or see light radiating from your heart throughout your body and beyond. Repeat the following phrases over and over again. Visualize what these words mean to you as you repeat them. Make yourself believe them, even if right now you don't think you can bring that belief into your everyday life. By affirming that you "are" the following things, you will send this positive signal to your brain, your heart, your soul, God, and the universe.

> My heart is open to love,
> My eyes are open to opportunities,
> And my soul is open to healing.

Every spiritual guru from Deepak Chopra M. D. to Neale Donald Walsch says the same thing: The universe responds to the power of "I Am." You need to get negativity out of your thinking because you live what you affirm in your thoughts. From now on, you need the strength to define yourself in the positive, because this is what will help you. You ARE beautiful, you ARE smart, you ARE happy, you ARE successful, you ARE lucky, and you ARE a badass. Tell yourself every day all the positive things that you are, whether they seem logical at that moment or not. Don't be afraid of anything—you have already lived through a lot, and fears will only get in the way of your success. Remember that you have unlimited potential, and that you will create yourself from this day forward.

Furthermore, if you ever catch yourself saying anything like "I am a failure," immediately replace that negative word within something positive. Two of my good friends have replaced the word "fat" with "fabulous!" Imagine the difference in energy between the phrases "I feel fat," and "I feel fabulous." Even though they know what they're saying, it changes the energy immediately. And of course, they burn a few calories just by laughing when they go shopping: "These ice cream sandwiches are too fabulous for us." "This soup has eight grams of saturated fabulous."

Always remember that you are a good person and that you are loved, even if it doesn't feel like it. Every day of your life involves choice: you can choose to focus on the negative, or you can accept that "this too shall pass," and accept the negative while you focus on the positive. You can take this experience to learn and grow from it. Although you might have more negativity right now than some of your friends do, after you have been through this hard time, you will see that every person in the world goes through a period of having dark times that can sometimes last for years. Every day that you get a little more control over yourself and your life is an important day in your spiritual evolution.

My Child, My Decisions
While you are pregnant, people will weigh in on your decisions without invitation: What to name the baby, whether to vaccinate or not, whether you plan to (or even can) breastfeed, whether to circumcise, whether your child will be going to daycare, etc. Depending on what your choices are, this may become insulting, domineering, or overwhelming, regardless of whether or not you are considering their input.

Selecting a Name
An area in which everyone will be all too quick to give opinions is in connection with choosing the baby's name. As a single mother who has decided on her own that this baby will have life, it is your sole privilege to name the baby whatever you like. Everybody will have their chance to name their own child. Only listen to *yourself* when it comes to naming your own.

But even more importantly, keep in mind that a single mother is *not obligated in any way to give her child its father's last name.* The tradition of using the father's last name is not a world-wide tradition and will also have no bearing on whether or not your child is entitled to child support from his or her natural father.

Even if the father of your child accepts paternity of your baby, it is still best for your autonomy to err on the side of caution and give the baby your own last name—after all, you're not married: he has no commitment to you, but you do have a commitment to the baby. In giving your baby your own last name, you will also avoid having to correct people who assume that you are Mrs. So-and-so (better to correct the Mrs. than the so-and-so), and you and your child will be given the privilege of sharing your surname as well as the possibility of passing on your family name.

And besides, if this man decides (like so many of them do) that he does not want to be a consistent part of his child's life, your child is going to wonder all his/her life who the heck this guy was, and why he was important enough to have the right to stamp his name on the child and then leave. Some people feel it's humiliating *not* to have your father's last name, but I think it would be ten times as humiliating to have the name of someone who is nowhere to be found, and rather alienating to have a different last name than everyone in your true family.

Additionally, based on my experience, American kids generally don't like having hyphenated names: They're just too long. Furthermore, it's difficult for people to figure out which one is the "real" surname (in some countries, it's the second one, but in our country, many people assume it's the first one). Also, have you ever had to fill out paperwork (customs and immigration forms, for example) in which you had to put one letter in each square, only to find that there weren't enough squares to fit the word you're intending to write?

If one day you choose to marry someone who is not the father of your baby and he wants to adopt your child, carefully consider whether or not you want to change your name, and make sure you allow your child to have a choice in the matter. I have personally seen many marriages come and go, but my son is going to be my son no matter what happens.

Be proud of your contribution to this child's life. This child is yours, nobody else's. At this time, you are this child's one and only real parent. Don't give away the exclusive privilege to name your child without a knock-down drag-out fight.

My personal decisions regarding other matters were constantly under fire throughout my pregnancy: Which vaccines to accept and which to reject, whether or not to circumcise my son, whether or not to sleep with a baby in the bed, whether to have a natural childbirth, etc.

Interestingly, I did make a commitment to have a natural birth, but it didn't quite work out that way—instead, I had a super pleasant forceps delivery because by the time I was in trouble, it was too late to have a C-section. So many people insist that it is possible for everyone to have a natural vaginal birth, but and while it may be ideal, shit happens! There is so much focus put on a woman's plans and intentions, and depending on your caregivers, there can be a lot of pressure to follow through with them. Some people I know feel guilt and inadequacy because of how their birth turned out. One birth author I'd dealt with for a short time insinuated that my birth would have been a lot easier if I'd been "more empowered." To that I say, "bullshit." My birth challenges were of a physical nature, as are those of women who ultimately have a C-section, planned or not.

Breastfeeding is also a hot topic. While it is true that breastfeeding is the healthiest, safest, most convenient, and most economical way to feed your baby (and is healthy for the mother too), the circumstances of new single mothers are so diverse that it is inadvisable for anyone to take a hard line on this topic. Our prevailing culture is not geared towards promoting the health of children and mothers, and being single imposes even more limitations on one's ability to follow through with their plans due to physical reasons (everyone's breasts are unique, not only in appearance, but also in function) (certain medications can be passed on through the mother's milk), emotional reasons (traumatic birth, lack of support), or economic reasons (having to return to work soon after the baby is born). In a perfect world, every mother would get the support that she needs in order to follow through with a commitment to breastfeed, and would be able to stay home with her baby for a year or more before returning to work without having to worry about her needs being met. Some countries are far ahead of the United States when it comes to understanding that a healthy start creates healthy people. But this is not currently a perfect world, and sometimes single mothers suffer judgment and condemnation for their failure to breastfeed, regardless of whether it's due to circumstances beyond their control.

While there is the resource of lactation/breastfeeding consultants, some mothers will tell you their stories of the line between support and pressure, as many such consultants have ultimately forsaken their subjects by refusing to internalize that all women who are trying to do what's best for their children need and deserve patience and understanding when trying to learn this important skill. Honestly, the good ones are very good, and are worth their weight in gold. But some breastfeeding campaigners have turned what would otherwise be committed natural mothers away from breastfeeding altogether by acting as though any deficiency or limitation is the fault and responsibility of the mother at an emotionally and physically trying time.

My dearest friend and I both experienced such extreme pressure from lactation consultants that neither of us achieved success in mastering this skill the first time around.

In my case, I was in extreme discomfort from having had a forceps delivery, and I was experiencing pain that I can compare to a sewing machine needle going into my breast because my son wasn't properly latching on. My mother was at a loss for how to help, as she hadn't experienced these complications, but the lactation consultant's impatience was angering me, as was the way she was handling my son's extremely bruised head. After I was told to quit making excuses and stop acting like a child, I excused *her*.

In the case of my dear friend, whose son had immediately gone into open heart surgery due to his heart valves closing improperly, the lactation consultants were demanding that she begin pumping her breasts while her son was on the operating table. She insisted that they leave her alone until she knew that her son would survive, as she was unsure as to whether these would be her last moments with her child (at this time I will note that he is both healthy and thriving), but they would not let up. She angrily sent them away. By the time her son was recovered from his surgery and she was able to hold him, she was no longer lactating.

By the time she had her second child, she was still battling feelings of anger towards these lactation consultants, but did manage to successfully breastfeed her daughter. Still, she refers to lactation consultants as "breastfeeding Nazis," and her success the second time around was achieved without their assistance.

Despite my bad experience and that of my friend (as well as scores of other women who have had similar experiences), I urge you to do your best to breastfeed, even if you are only able to breastfeed for a short time. But rather than make breastfeeding imperative, I will honor your unique circumstances and perspective by offering strategies for minimizing the risks of formula feeding in the event that it becomes necessary.

Bottles: Make sure any bottles you use are free of Bisphenol A, a highly toxic synthetic estrogen hormone that has been found to promote reproductive impacts, cancer, obesity, and miscarriage. If you are unsure whether your bottles contain this toxic hormone, e-mail or write to the company and ask. In the event that they try to convince you that their bottles are safe despite using Bisphenol A, stay away from those bottles.

Water: All water used to make formula should be purified water (do not mistake distilled water for purified water). Invest in a water purifier to use with tap water or well water, but don't use your public water at all if your community has known or suspected water problems. While I don't recommend bottled water for many reasons (some brands are simply purified tap water anyway), there is no way to adequately purify the public water in some communities. In this instance, it is preferred that you purchase drinking water in jugs for use in the home, and please recycle. The water you use for formula must be warm, but not hot. If you test the stream of water on your wrist, it should feel neither warm nor cold.

Formula: Even some pediatricians are unaware that the growth hormone fed to many of our nation's dairy cows (rBST or rBGH) appears in baby formula at 500 times the amount at which it was tested for human safety when it met with FDA approval. In addition, the tested sample was pasteurized at much higher heat than is used on any of our dairy products. For this reason, many formula companies claim that all of the growth hormone is destroyed in the pasteurization process, which is simply untrue: *None of it* is destroyed in the pasteurization process.

Some mothers believe that they can bypass these risks by feeding their children soy formula, and some mothers opt for soy formula due to allergies or other health concerns. However, non-organic soy is often genetically engineered and has pesticides and herbicides built right into its genes. As a result, it is more dangerous than rBST. With soy formula, it is every bit as important to use *only* organic formula.

Furthermore, even organic soy formula carries its own set of risks due to trypsin inhibitors, phytic acid, which inhibit absorption of nutrients, and phytoestrogens, which can negatively affect a baby's hormone balance, causing retarded growth of a boy's sex organs, and early reproductive development or fertility problems later in life for females.

Therefore, while some people have diminished choice in the matter, special care must go into the decision of what to feed an infant if the mother can't breastfeed.

Thankfully, our nation is waking up to this food safety crisis, but it is your responsibility to stay one step ahead of the game until the laws and regulations are changed for the better. If you use formula, use only organic formula. This will minimize your child's chances of suffering from any of the diseases and conditions that are linked to exposure to rBST and GMO soy, including allergies and pancreatic cancer. Organic formula is expensive, and is sometimes very hard to find in some areas, but in the long run is well worth the expense, as it is better to invest in your baby's health now rather than having to manage allergies, asthma, and any other conditions that may arise from exposing your baby to unnecessary hormones and toxins.

As a final word: these choices are yours. I can encourage you to do your research and share my knowledge, but in so doing, I do not hope to make you feel as though you need to defend your personal reasons for your own choices, as your energy needs to go towards more important things right now. Whatever your heart (and extensive research) is telling you to do, do exactly that. You have every right to make these decisions. If people don't agree with your choices, they can exercise these decisions on their own children, *not yours*!

Gratitude for what is Yours

Just as you will probably experience extremely pessimistic influences while you are pregnant, you will also most likely have friends, co-workers, and relatives who are enthusiastic about your undertaking and who will provide their emotional support and bolster your courage throughout this potentially difficult time. Those people who are helping you through these times deserve some recognition and consideration for a job well done.

Following is a list of rules for maintaining good relations with good people and letting them know that they have been a big help.

#1: Do not rely too much on one person. Although you may be closer to one person than all the others, remember that your life is not their responsibility. Commissioning your best friend to have involvement in each and every one of your tasks may make him or her feel as though they have somehow wound up in a marriage of inconvenience without the sex. It is okay to ask for a favor every now and then, but don't be hurt if you don't have someone holding your hand through every doctor visit. Your *very* best friend should always be yourself.

#2: Do not take advantage of a friend or family member's generosity. The people in your life may be going on a bit of a buying spree for you, and yes, you probably need some TLC. But remember that every relationship needs balance, and that if you don't give back, the gravy train just might jump the tracks. Always acknowledge those friends and relatives who are giving you help. Give greeting cards. Cook special dinners at home. If a friend gives you baby clothes, promise to give them a photograph of their outfit after your baby is born. This will show your loved ones that you care even if you're not in the financial shape to match them dollar for dollar.

#3: Return positivity with positivity. Nobody enjoys beating their head against a wall. Do not counter every positive statement with "Yeah, but…" or "You just don't understand." Reward your loved ones for their positive attitude by returning it. Don't drag anybody down. If during a conversation you feel that you are too down to be up, let your loved one know that you're in a funk and feel that you are incapable of providing good company at the moment. Promise to get back in touch with them when you are feeling better, and do something solitary and productive like meditating, writing poetry, organizing your closet, or devising ways of making more money.

#4: Remember that you are not the only person in the world who needs attention. Be a good listener to your good friends. Sure, you may not be able to relate to your friend's problem of having to choose between two enviable eligible bachelors or her concerns about gaining too much weight, but her problems are just as big in her life as your problems are in yours. Give her the consideration she has given you, and someday you'll be able to bore her with comparable trivial problems and hopefully she'll be there for you!

#5. Realize that there is no such thing as the right or wrong time to have a baby: You're having a baby, and that's fantastic! A woman's biological clock isn't something that can be easily negotiated with. When I was pregnant, I was envious of many of my friends who continued to have physical autonomy and financial freedom. Sometimes they would say things like, "for us, it's not the right time." They were being "responsible" and waiting until they were "ready." Sometimes, that made me feel rather stupid. But twelve years later, many of those friends were stuck at home with their babies and toddlers, and were wishing they could go out. Others are trying very hard to have babies, and aren't having any luck.

One single friend got accidentally pregnant at the age of 41. Without a partner as she was, she was excited to have her first and only baby. She'd been working successfully as a hairdresser for almost 20 years (most of those years with her own studio), so she didn't have to worry about fitting an education or career plan into her life as a parent. However, she too fielded comments about her timeline. "Aren't you worried that the baby is going to have Down's syndrome?" "You're going to be 60 years old when the baby graduates from high school." "You will never retire." It seems that no matter when you have a baby, some people think it's wrong. The solution: Be happy and ignore all that.

If your friends' or strangers' comments about your age or time line make you feel like you are doing something wrong, remember that if anyone expects their entire life to go as they had planned, they are in for a big surprise some day.

People are the most important blessings in our lives, and these blessings should be counted every day, whether your method consists of putting a reminder on your refrigerator or including your loved ones in your nightly prayers or meditations. If you feel as though you don't have the love and support of enough people, reach out to others in your church, your support group, your neighborhood, or your extended family. Give thanks that you live in America where you likely have clean water and a bed to sleep in, and not a third-world country where you have to dig through the dump to find food or something to sell. Take time to read *The Grapes of Wrath*, and acknowledge that life in this country did not always provide the opportunities you now have. Find inspiration in all that is positive in your life ranging from the profound (my mother, my health, etc.) to the superficial (my furniture, my long eyelashes…). Focus on what's right in your life (you may find that you have more to be thankful for than you thought), and work towards correcting that which you feel could use improvement. Remember that the most important person in your life, the one who will truly be there to help you through the bad times is *you*, so be as easy on yourself as you can be.

Do Not "Let Yourself Go!"

Yes, we've all seen that poor haggard woman, haunting the grocery store like a moldering cadaver, staring at her feet as she slumps down the aisles: We've seen the greasy hair, the sagging sweats, the stained t-shirt, the bags beneath her eyes, and the countenance that says "I just don't care anymore." True, there is nothing wrong with what she's doing, and her lack of enthusiasm might even have been a result of her husband's convincing her that there's no point in looking good, so why even try? Married with children and (as many perceive her to be) "past her prime," she may feel she's got no one to impress.

You, on the other hand, have everyone to impress. After all, you have a responsibility not only to other single mothers, but also to your child, to embody self-respect and to promote yourself and do whatever's necessary to knock down the hurdles that stand between you and the perfect life you and your child deserve. People who show respect for their appearance are treated better in public (which always helps with the attitude) and are more quickly promoted at work, regardless of whether or not they possess natural beauty. You don't have to be a beauty queen, you don't have to be in perfect shape, and you don't have to have beautiful clothes in order to exhibit self-respect. You cannot, however, let yourself go. Maintaining your appearance and sense of style is like putting on your suit of armor to deflect harm from your adversaries. In the event that you feel you are one of the few who can pull off a T-shirt-and-sweatpants grocery run, do keep in mind that you can find a t-shirt free of stains at the Salvation Army for fifty cents. You *can* be comfortable and still be proud.

And despite our culture's short-sighted belief that a woman maintains her appearance solely for the purpose of attracting suitors (which turns a woman's personal pride into a desperate cry for company), rest assured that this is another cultural tactic designed to keep your hands out of the cookie jar of success. Although sexual opportunity is one of many reasons to look your best, I'm sure my neighbor's neutered dog wasn't thinking about his sexuality when his owner shaved him for the summer and he hid behind the couch for a week. Your body is an extension of your personality—use it as a canvas to show the world who you are. You don't do yourself or anyone else any good by hiding your light from the world you are meant to conquer.

Of course any changes to your physical appearance should be on your own terms, and don't be overly self-critical about things you can't control, such as the weight gain or stretch marks that are suffered by most pregnant women. Furthermore, opinions vary widely concerning whether make-up really does make a woman look better or if it simply makes her look made-up, whether a modern haircut looks better than one-length hair, etc. But there are some standards that most everyone can agree on: People look their best in clean clothes, clean hair, and skin as healthy as it can get.

You can help assure that your body and skin stay as healthy as possible during your pregnancy by eating well, engaging in moderate exercise, drinking enough water, and taking your prenatal vitamins. Eat natural meats (free of hormones and antibiotics) if you can afford them (this is especially important with ground beef), eat organic fruits and vegetables whenever they are available, and drink organic milk if you can afford it, as antibiotics, growth hormones, and pesticides all contribute to unnecessary weight gain, bad skin, and health problems for you and possibly the baby as well. Try to reduce your sodium. The FDA's recommended daily allowance is based on bad science. If you keep your sodium below 1500 milligrams a day, you are in great shape. Stay *away* from the fast food. It will clog your arteries, tax your liver, discolor your skin, and pack on the unnecessary pounds. Make no mistake about it: fast food is *not* food: its value is in being able to take the edge off if you're extremely hungry, but don't perceive it as real food.

Taking a half-hour walk three times a week will not only provide your body with exercise, but will also give you just enough sun exposure to clear up your skin and give you some color without over-exposing yourself. Your body needs the sun in order to make vitamin D, so you don't have to hide from the sun all the time—you just have to use common sense.

As far as your wardrobe is concerned, if anything has stains on it, cut it into pieces and use it as rags unless you really do use those shirts for painting or gardening. Sure, the stained clothes thing might be kind of cute if you're twelve, but on a pregnant woman, unless she is painting or gardening, it just looks bad. Even the clothes that you wear to slouch around the house in should be garments that wouldn't cause you shame in the event that you have to make a late-night run to the market. Your pregnancy does not in and of itself make you unsightly, nor does it make you invisible. It is indeed your choice whether you want to be viewed as someone who cares about herself or someone who has completely given up. You may not feel your best right now, but you cannot give up on yourself, as every single pregnant woman who stands proud in the face of society's judgment can help change our world's perception of women.

Start Preventing Postpartum Depression NOW
These days, there is a medication meant to address any malady that can strike a person, including depression. As one who has seen many women suffer from postpartum depression, I have witnessed many a psychological emergency that needed immediate attention. As a steadfast advocate of single pregnant women, I would never judge any woman for taking anti-depressant medications in order to keep herself sane and her child safe, but the fact remains that too many anti-depressant medications have potentially dangerous side effects, some of them even more severe than the depression itself.

Often times it takes a few days to a few weeks in order for the patient's brain to adjust to the prescribed medication, putting the patient on an emotional roller-coaster until her body chemistry settles into the changes that relieve the depression. Sometimes the patient's body rejects the medication all together, and the medication causes a more severe depression than that which was originally being addressed. However, sometimes the medications work right away, work well, and immediately provide relief for the patient. The awful truth is that one never knows until she tries.

Again, keep in mind that drastic measures sometimes need to be taken when a pregnant woman or mother is in a state of emergency. However, if one is not currently in a state of emergency, it is important that she takes measures to keep it that way.

These days, anti-depressants (as well as other types of medications) are carelessly over-prescribed. Some doctors get kick-backs (special incentives such as vacations) for prescribing a medication. Although it is possible to find a doctor who works from her heart and wants to do right by her patients regardless of any potential awards, many doctors got into the business for status and money. Once upon a time, medicine and law were the two professions in which a person was guaranteed a large income, and doctors who are motivated primarily by money will feel that your actual health is of no consequence when a trip to Hawaii is on the line (we'll get into lawyers later).

Another thing one must consider about western medicine is that doctors are taught to fix problems through drugs and surgery rather than through natural means. We can't really judge them for not knowing the inexpensive and natural ways to treat maladies when all of their schooling, study, and indoctrination has been focused on drugs and surgery. Granted, a doctor can repair a broken leg better than any other type of professional, but we must ask ourselves this: If a person is depressed, what exactly has been broken? Is it a broken heart? A broken spirit? These things cannot be fixed through drugs or surgery, and certainly cannot be addressed in the event that this body has not be running on the proper fuel. Many people do legitimately have a "chemical imbalance," but often times that chemical imbalance can be a direct result of their body's reaction to what they've been ingesting. For example, the combination of Aspartame (in most diet sodas) and MSG (a flavor enhancer found in products including Doritos) can inhibit brain function, resulting inability to concentrate, depression, and more. The FDA is perfectly aware of the fact that this combination is harmful and does not approve food products which contain both these ingredients together, but the information about the potential harmful effects of this combination are not readily available to the public. When a doctor is interviewing a patient about their depression, how many doctors ask the question, "So, have you been eating Doritos and drinking diet soda together?" When it comes to addressing depression and other ailments, many Americans believe that to take a medication is their best course of action, but is it really? Sure, the symptoms of these problems once someone is in a state of emergency can sometimes be addressed and corrected, but wouldn't it be better if they could be stopped at the source?

For a short while, I took an antidepressant called Welbutrin, also known as Zyban, to help me quit smoking. Although I wasn't exactly happy before I started taking the Welbutrin, seven days after I started taking it, I was a whimpering, miserable, blubbering mess who couldn't have a conversation without crying and could hardly get out of bed. In addition, I started getting migraines for the first (and last) time in my life, and even started sleepwalking. It took three days from the time I stopped taking the drug to the time I could go through a day without crying or feeling like I was going to die. For a single mother with an infant, three days can be a very long time to endure these feelings.

There's another useful personal anecdote that's a bit embarrassing, as I would never have found myself in the position to need emergency psychological intervention if I had simply taken better care of myself through meditation, rest, and simply learning not to over-commit myself, but this story has merit when it comes to demonstrating how our nation's medical culture doesn't always do right by us. On this occasion, I was going through a very stressful time in my life when I needed intermittent relief for occasional extreme anxiety. After talking to my friends, I found that Xanax is what is normally prescribed, and I asked my nurse practitioner for a prescription for Xanax. My nurse practitioner agreed to give me the Xanax, but only if I agreed to try an antidepressant called Paxil as well, which I was to take every day and was expected to "kick in" within about six weeks. I told her that my anxiety, although severe, was only intermittent and I didn't need to be on a daily regimen that would alter my brain chemistry to the point of my needing to commit to a drug that I would eventually have to wean myself from. In addition, my anxiety was related to a friend's going in to brain surgery soon, a court custody battle, and a work project with an ex-boyfriend, all of which were to be over within six weeks. I had heard many things about Paxil, some of it good but mostly bad: I'd heard that often it made people lazy, increased their depression, made them eat constantly, and took a long time to leave one's system. My nurse practitioner didn't budge. It was either both or neither. I paid for my office visit, and walked away empty-handed. Embarrassingly, I didn't think to take both prescriptions and fill just the Xanax prescription, but those kinds of things happen when you're distracted!

The next day, a friend gave me three of his own Xanax, warning me of all the side effects, and telling me to take half a pill if my anxiety got unbearable. When I took that Xanax, I knew it was the right thing to do: It reminded my body of how it felt to be calm, and it helped me remember what to "aim for" when my anxiety was approaching. I only took two more half-pills within the next few weeks, which completely got me through my crisis. That was all I needed: one and a half pills. I did not need, nor did I want, nor could

I use a six-week prescription to an anti-depressant, but that's what I (thought I) had to agree to in order to get my relief from a "legitimate" medical professional!

Based on my personal experience and that of many friends and acquaintances, my opinion is this: *Increasing your body's level of toxicity is rarely the best way to prevent, or combat depression!*

Yes, drugs can be used as a last resort to TREAT depression, but many factors that set the stage for developing depression can be prevented through educating yourself, eating healthy foods, getting moderate exercise, and practicing meditation, prayer, or positive affirmations on a regular basis. Unlike drugs, there is *no risk* in increasing your physical, mental, and emotional health naturally. Do not be too hard on yourself if you are already in a state of psychological emergency (like I was when I needed the Xanax), but do take initiative in making yourself as healthy as possible, starting now.

In order to assure that your overall health is in tip-top shape for the potential pressures of new parenthood, this is what you need to do:

Educate yourself on nutrition
With the very toxic eating habits we Americans have, combined with the corruption of the FDA and USDA, it's hard to tell what is and isn't healthy these days. If you buy a bottle of Sunny Delight, you may think you're drinking orange juice, when in fact you are drinking mostly high fructose corn syrup, the ingredient most responsible for America's obesity and Type 2 diabetes epidemics, and less than 2 percent fruit juice. You may think that applesauce is a healthy snack for you *and* for your baby, but non-organic applesauce often contains up to 90 known carcinogens due to the pesticides used on apples. You may have heard of soy products as an alternative to dairy, but are unaware that most non-organic soy in this country is genetically engineered, has never been tested for safety in the United States, and has been found to kill unborn rats when their mothers were fed genetically engineered soy in tests performed in Russia. Many protein shakes, even those sold in natural food stores, are made with non-organic soy protein, so that's definitely something to watch for!

According to Dharma Singh Khalsa, author of *Food as Medicine*, we can increase our physical AND mental health by addressing the level of toxicity in our bodies. As one who had started eating organic foods and clean proteins due mainly to political rather than health reasons, I was happy to see my philosophy echoed by a strong medical authority such as Dr. Khalsa, and I was even happier to notice the unexpected physical and emotional changes in my body after changing the way I ate. I highly recommend this book to any human being who eats, but in summary, you will be healthier both physically and mentally if you eat organic foods, and many mental and physical health issues can be addressed simply by eating the right things.

We all understand that when you're pregnant, your body sometimes dictates what one's stomach can tolerate. I say go ahead and have that hamburger you crave, but it's best if you can make it with organic or naturally processed, grass-fed ground beef, a sprouted grain bun, organic lettuce, tomatoes, and condiments. Go ahead and have the hot dog, but make sure it's either organic, or ideally, a great tasting organic meat-free hot dog! Eliminating pesticides, growth hormones, and genetically engineered ingredients from your diet may not seem to have a short-term effect, but your mood, health, and weight, and that of your child, will all be subtly (if not profoundly) affected by these changes to your diet.

Eat healthy foods
Yes, after the last paragraph you are probably a bit overwhelmed. Who knew that there were demons hiding in the angels of nutrition? It's really not fair to any of us, especially those of us who are on such a tight budget that buying all organic foods seems unrealistic at the moment. BUT even if you are not ready to go organic, there are a few things you can do to maximize your nutrition within your budget, which will positively affect your mental and emotional health as well.

Drink truly clean water
Every household should have a water filter, as many toxic chemicals are in our water supplies, regardless of whether our water comes from the city or a well. A water filter can be obtained from practically any supermarket in the United States.

Forget all about fast food
As I've said before and will say again, fast food is *not* food! If indeed fast food does taste good to you, it will stop tasting good as soon as you watch the documentary *Supersize Me* or read *Fast Food Nation*, or *Mad Cow USA*. In short, fast food is not meant to sustain life, it's meant to take it away at a profit to someone else.

Fast food is designed through laboratory-created smells to trick your brain into thinking it's food when indeed it is no such thing, and also tricks your body into continuing to eat after you are full. It fills your stomach without providing any nutrition, taxes your liver, clogs your colon, clogs your arteries, and if you eat it too much, it can kill you. And if that's not enough to turn you off, go out right now and get yourself your LAST Burger King Whopper. Eat the whole thing, wash your hands for about five seconds, dry them, and then smell them. Did you get the smell off? Wash them again. How about now? That smell lingers because it is not the natural scent of meat, lettuce, tomatoes, ketchup, mayonnaise, cheese, and a bun, but is instead a synthetic scent that is added to your food, and is meant to beckon you from far away. Smell them again. Take a big whiff. And think about it.

If you make hamburgers, tacos, or hot dogs at home, they may still be fattening, but they will at least provide you with some nutrition. Do not support the evil fast food industry, because they are not supporting anyone but themselves.

Kick the soda habit

This decision can make a huge impact on your health and life. If you are a Coke-a-day girl like I used to be, this may seem like shutting the door on your best friend. But any soda, be it diet or non-diet, is not your best friend, it's an enemy that betrays your health every day.

Diet sodas often contain highly-toxic engineered sugar substitutes (most recently Aspartame, marketed as "Nutrasweet," and Sucralose, sold as Splenda) that are never sufficiently tested for safety before they're put on the shelves.

Products that contain Stevia, if they don't also contain fillers, are safe—Stevia has been used as a natural sweetener all over the world for centuries with no negative health effects, yet it was under fire by the FDA for being unsafe as a sweetener, although it was approved as a supplement. Later, there was some circulating propaganda that suggested that it is not safe for pregnant women, despite never having been tested to reach this conclusion. To make a long story short, we now *know* that Aspartame and Sucralose *are* unsafe, yet they remain as an additive in many food products. Many thanks, FDA, for protecting us from the bad guys (yes, I am being sarcastic)!

At one time, Aspartame was owned by Monsanto chemical company, the same company responsible for such poisons as DDT, Agent Orange, and Roundup weed killer. Interestingly Monsanto sold aspartame to another company—a food additive that has been proven to cause a variety of health problems (including pancreas cancer) was too much of a liability even for a company that specialized in creating and marketing products that kill. If being skinny is worth destroying your health, keep drinking. Approximately six months after your death, you'll be as thin as a bone!

The other dirty contender on the sweetener scene is Sucralose, branded as Splenda. Exercise caution when using this stuff. Like Aspartame, it is made from chemicals. It was actually discovered in 1976 by scientists in the UK who were seeking a new pesticide formulation, and is made by replacing hydroxyl groups in the sugar molecule with chlorine! At the time of this writing, there have been no long-term studies on the side effects of using Sucralose, but the maker's own short-term studies have shown shrunken thymus glands and enlarged livers and kidneys in laboratory rats.

Non-diet sodas normally contain high fructose corn syrup (HFCS) which is in just about everything, and is just plain BAD. Since the American public started catching on to the health risks of HFCS, now food companies are marketing the same substance as "fructose," which has traditionally been understood to be a natural product, or "fructose syrup."

Some products that use HFCS are now using labels that say "Does not contain HFCS!" But then when you read the label, the ingredient "fructose syrup" is listed, which is the same thing. Many savvy consumers believe that the use of the term "fructose" is to manipulate people into believing that this chemical-bathed, hyper-sweetened garbage is in fact a healthy alternative to sugar. The fact is that it is simply cheaper, and that the rates of both Type 2 Diabetes and obesity have skyrocketed since our country was converted to the overuse of this cheap and dangerous sweetener. And yes, they duped us all. At this time, this sweetener is in salad dressings, ketchup, soups, sodas, sauces, and even bread!

Although refined white sugar is not exactly healthy, it is a much healthier choice than what is currently labeled as fructose. However, sparsely tested genetically modified sugar beets have now been approved for inclusion in non-organic foods that contain sugar. Please note that cane sugar is not genetically modified, and some of the most popular brands of sugar are now adding "non-GMO" to their labels because they want to make sure that food savvy people (like you) will know they are not GMO.

If eliminating sodas seems too difficult right now, downgrade the toxicity of your soda by switching to a soda without caffeine, without caramel color, and that uses evaporated cane juice rather than HFCS, fructose, or fructose syrup. Ginger Ale is a good choice. Not only is it less toxic than Coke or Pepsi, but the ginger settles the stomach, and many pregnant women like it for this reason.

If you are a diet soda drinker, there are a few options available to you: Start drinking iced tea or sodas sweetened with Stevia or Xylitol. Tea comes in many flavors and some types boast health benefits. When shopping for diet sodas, look in the natural foods section of your supermarket, and avoid anything that contains aspartame (in Nutrasweet) or the newest offender, Sucralose (in Splenda). Also keep in mind that if/when you get used to it, nothing is healthier and more risk-free than a glass of plain water with lemon.

Know what's in your juice

Anyone who was alive in the eighties remembers that you could never assume that a beverage that looked like orange juice was in fact orange juice. It could have been Tang, which was mostly sugar, or it could have been Sunny Delight, which was also mostly sugar. The only way to know the truth was to take a taste, and sometimes what was tasted was an unpleasant surprise. Other products were also referred to as "juice": Kool-Aid, Capri Sun, and Hawaiian Punch. When it started to become apparent that these beverages were predominantly sugar, it ushered in some healthier-looking health impostors: Sports drinks, energy drinks, flavored waters, and smoothies with just as much sugar as the fake juices. One might think that a smoothie is healthier than having a piece of cake with ice cream, but if it's a smoothie that is prepared by anyone other than you, it might not be. Sadly, even 100 percent fruit juice contains a lot of sugar, but it is more easily metabolized if it's the sugar that naturally grows within fruit, and it will provide the benefits of real nutrition.

That said, if you drink juice at all, never waste your time, your money, or the space in your stomach for any juice that's not either 100 percent fruit juice. If for some reason you ever stray from 100 percent fruit juice, at least make sure it's naturally sweetened, and think of said beverage as a "treat:" you are hydrating your body and enjoying the flavor, but you will get your nutrition later.

Know the "dirty (baker's) dozen"
Although pesticides are always bad for the environment, some non-organic (conventionally grown) crops are worse than others for your body, due to the fact that they absorb more pesticides than do other plants. This list changes every few years, so I am going beyond the dirty dozen and including all contenders that have been on this list since I started paying attention. It is not in everyone's budget to buy organic, but for the sake of your health, try to buy organic when purchasing these products:

- Strawberries
- Apples & apple products
- Celery
- Spinach
- Bell Peppers
- Cherries
- Nectarines
- Peaches
- Pears
- Potatoes
- Red Raspberries
- Green Beans
- Cucumbers
- Grapes
- Tomatoes

Know which produce is low in pesticide contamination
There are also some items that remain safe and healthy despite conventional farming methods. These include:

- Avocadoes
- Pineapples

Cabbage
Onions
Asparagus
Mangoes
Papayas
Kiwis
Eggplant
Honeydew Melon
Grapefruit
Cantaloupe
Cauliflower
Sweet Potatoes

Avoid GMOs (Genetically Modified Organisms)

Genetically Modified Organisms, or GMOs, are ingredients usually made from plants whose genes have been altered to include pesticides, pesticide resistance, resistance to cold or disease, etc. You (or more likely your parents, as most of those of us who were adults at the time are no longer having kids) may remember the FlavrSavr tomato which was bred with a flounder (yes, that is a fish) so that it could withstand cold temperatures. Thankfully, due to a mushy consistency and short shelf live, the FlavrSavr was pulled from the market in 1997.

GMO foods are produced by powerful chemical companies, and it seems that the American public never catches on to these companies' agendas until it is too late. One of the reasons High Fructose Corn Syrup is so popular is because it is made by Monsanto chemical company, which wields a lot of power. Indeed they do have enough power to get FDA and USDA approval for products that are in no way safe, but they will never have the power to prevent you from finding out the truth about their products, refusing to consume them, and voting with your dollars!

Believe it or not, limiting GMO foods can be easy once you learn a few avoidance strategies! Of course, the easiest avoidance strategy is to buy and eat organic because organic foods do not contain GMOs. But if you can't go 100 percent organic, your next line of defense is to avoid non-organic foods that contain any products made from GMO crops. At the time of this writing, all you have to do is avoid all non-organic corn, cottonseed, soy, canola, papaya, squash, and sugar beet products—and there are two brand new GMO food items to watch for: "White Russet" potatoes and "Arctic" apples.

Of course, learning which products are made from these crops is tricky because food products and additives change and have misleading names, but it is often possible if you avoid anything non-organic with soy, corn, cottonseed, or canola in their names (soy isolates, cornmeal, cottonseed oil, etc.). Another GMO avoidance strategy to be used in restaurants is to ask if the oil used in preparing foods is non-organic canola. If it is, request that your foods be prepared with olive oil or butter. While this helps you to avoid GMOs, it also communicates to the restaurant that it is important for you to avoid GMOs, which can sometimes prompt an establishment to change their recipes. Although the wind may change (and Monsanto chemical company has a track record of staying one step ahead of consumer knowledge), beat them at their own game by avoiding anything you know is genetically modified, and stay informed. Knowing what is really in your food will honestly change the way you eat from this day forward.

Limit caffeine

If you have a habit of drinking coffee, tea, or soda, now is the time to get that habit under control. Yes, at this time coffee is "fashionable," but at one time it was also fashionable to smoke. Caffeine, like nicotine, is a drug. Have you ever noticed how angry and aggressive some people can be before they've had their first cup of morning coffee? Have you ever noticed how nothing feels quite right after you've had *too much* coffee in one day? It makes you nervous, irritable, and generally dissatisfied with life. Imagine how a breastfeeding baby might feel after having fed on your milk laced with coffee.

If your coffee habit is simply too much to let go, start cutting the dose with decaf. If you like specialty coffee drinks, start asking for half-caff until you get used to the taste, but also consider that a "specialty coffee drinks" habit can be rather costly! Breaking this habit will benefit not only your health, but your bank account as well.

Know what's in your meat

Although American citizens are starting to wake up to the fact that conventionally processed meats present significant health risks through the irresponsible use of antibiotics and hormones, many Americans are still unaware that the United States is the only "civilized" country that fails to adhere to World Health Organization standards for the prevention of and testing for Mad Cow Disease, and practices standards that allow various resistant viruses and bacteria, including Listeria and E Coli 0157, to flourish. Americans are also often shocked to find out what causes Mad Cow Disease: Cannibalism. To save money, most factory farms feed blood (rather than milk) to calves, which is a cause of Mad Cow Disease. Our country is in denial about our potential for having an extremely tainted meat supply because our country refuses to test sufficiently to find Mad Cow Disease in our cattle while continuing to feed blood to calves. Even more frightening is the fact that prions, the proteins caused by this cannibalism, can't be destroyed through radiation, incineration, freezing, or any known drug. If you burry prions in the soil, that soil will still hold infectivity many years later. Prions are not specific to any species—cow prions will have the same effect on humans—the rise of Alzheimer's disease and other degenerative disorders should be looked at much more closely. At the time of this writing, there is no known way to destroy prions, aside from autoclaving them or dousing them with extremely fresh bleach.

The most potentially dangerous meat on the market is ground beef. Some of you might remember when tons of meat was recalled all over the west coast because one cow was found to have Mad Cow Disease. That's because thousands of cows, many of whom were too sick to walk (and were never tested for Mad Cow Disease), went through the offending slaughterhouse's grinder before our sloppy food safety standards required that it be cleaned. When you are eating ground beef that was ground in a typical meat processing plant, you are eating the meat of over a thousand cattle. Yuck.

If you like beef, make sure your ground beef is both organic, preferably organic *and* grass-fed. Companies that adhere to the standards required by these labels cannot improperly irradiate, medicate, or feed their cattle. Beef that is grass fed has more beneficial B vitamins than grain-fed beef, and has way less fat (you can lose several pounds a year by simply replacing your grain-fed beef with grass-fed beef). An extra bonus: Grass-fed beef is much better for the environment, as these farmers have no need to dump animal waste into our waterways.

Sadly, non-organic grass-fed beef in our county is often fed GMO alfalfa, the long-term health effects of which we cannot be certain, and the environmental impact of which is undeniably tragic.

Use high standards for pork and chicken as well. Look for pork that is organic or at least free of hormones and antibiotics, and chicken that is natural, organic, and/or free range.

Also, stay away from "gas-packed" meats (those with the cellophane wrapper that does not come into contact with the meat), even if they are labeled organic. Although the organic label prevents these companies from using carbon monoxide (a common practice in non-organic gas-packed meats) in their packing, all gas-packed meats are pumped full of sodium in order to keep them looking fresh past their spoilage dates, which can have negative health effects on those who are watching their sodium intake.

Thankfully, naturally processed meats can now be found in most markets across the country. True, organic and naturally processed meat is more expensive than conventionally fed and processed meat, but we Americans eat much more meat than is healthy anyway. If you upgrade your meat, you may begin to consume less of it, which will likely benefit your health.

Another way to avoid the toxins in our meat supply is to purchase or hunt wild game. Although there is an occasional exception, wild animals often have diets and live in environments that are far less toxic than animals who live and eat in factory farm feedlots.

Know what's in your milk/ dairy products
Most milk in the United States contains a hormone called Recombinant Bovine Growth Hormone (rBST or rBGH), which is injected into the cows to make them produce more milk. The health effects of this hormone at the levels that they appear in our milk have never been tested by independent researchers (researchers who don't have a relationship with the company that makes the hormone), and when it was tested, it was tested at 1/500th the level that this hormone occurs in our milk supply, and was pasteurized at 500 degrees for fifteen minutes, which is far hotter and far longer than any milk is *ever* pasteurized! We don't yet know of the exact health risks of these hormones, but we know that their purpose is to make cows larger and interfere with the natural functions of their endocrine systems. It makes sense that it might do the same to us human beings.

Make sure the milk (and other dairy products, including cheese and sour cream) you consume is free of this hormone. Although organic dairies are not allowed to use this hormone, these days there are plenty of non-organic dairies that refuse to use it as well. Thankfully, these days milk that is free of rBGH is often labeled.

Eat Your Omega-3 Fatty Acids
A growing fetus needs Omega-3 fatty acids. If a pregnant woman doesn't get enough of them, the fetus will take all there is, setting the stage for depression in the mother. A new mother can help prevent postpartum depression by making sure she has consumed enough of the following foods:

- Walnuts
- Salmon
- Herring
- Halibut
- Tuna (not recommended while you are pregnant due to mercury content)
- Grass-fed Beef
- Venison
- Buffalo
- Canola Oil (organic)
- Flaxseed and flaxseed oil
- Fish Oil capsules
- Omega-3 enriched eggs
- Omega-3 enriched mayonnaise

Eat Foods Rich in Folic Acid

Folic Acid is also part of a healthy diet for pregnant women. Folic Acid is an important component in maintaining your child's health, and a folic acid deficiency in your body can manifest itself in headaches, behavior disorders, exhaustion, diarrhea, and irritability, all of which can affect your mental health in both the short and long term. Both while you are pregnant and after, make sure you are eating the following foods:

> Oranges, orange juice
> Chickpeas, garbanzo beans, hummus
> Broccoli (raw or steamed)
> Peas
> Strawberries
> Collard greens
> Asparagus
> Lentils
> Papaya (Organic)

Decrease Your Dependency on Over-the-Counter Drugs

Many Americans are simply in the habit of taking an over-the-counter medication when they are ill, can't sleep, or simply don't feel very well. However, even over-the-counter medicines can be risky if taken improperly, taken too often, or taken with other over-the-counter medications. As a pregnant woman, you probably know by now that you must avoid ibuprofen at all costs, even though some people take ibuprofen on a daily basis. As a parent, you will learn that aspirin can be deadly to children who have the flu. In addition, the FDA is often under pressure from pharmaceutical companies to approve medications before they have been sufficiently tested (some may remember when Thera-flu was recalled because it was found that a main ingredient caused brain bleeding in children). Even if you are following all the precautions of an over-the-counter medicine, ALL medicines affect your liver and your immune system, and some of the ingredients in pharmaceuticals are so filthy that they're not even considered safe for inclusion in pet food. The medicines you find on the shelf of the grocery store can eliminate symptoms, but they can't make you well. Remember that the pharmaceutical industry, like the fast food industry, is based on money. It is designed to make a profit off providing comfort for you.   How they affect your health is really of no concern to them.

When you have a pain or ailment, try to consider the *source* of the ailment rather than simply putting a quick-fix over your pain.   You can often safely avoid a cold by drinking green tea with Echinacea at the first signs of illness, or by boiling an onion and ten cloves of garlic in water for 20 minutes, straining out the solids, mixing the water with lemon juice and honey, and drinking it. The best way to avoid getting any illness is through getting enough sleep, eating the right foods, washing your hands, dressing appropriately for the weather (wearing gloves can really cut down of the germs picked up by your hands), and being cautious about what you touch when in public areas.

Be smart and creative about how you address and combat your aches, pains, and illnesses. Don't take medicine for any ailment if the source of your problem can be traced to the food you eat. For example, if you're prone to getting acid indigestion, try eating more foods that are high in alkaline to decrease your dependency on antacids. The fewer toxic substances that are in your body (including medicines), the healthier and happier you'll be.

How do you do *That*?
"Really, I would love to be able to eat only the healthiest foods, but let's be real: How the heck am I supposed to be able to pull this off? I'm about to be a single mother for Christ's sake—Organic food is extremely expensive!"

Ah yes, the million dollar question: And yes, I have a solution.

Upon my graduation from college, my mom bought me what I have found to be the single most useful book I have ever owned. It's called *Where's Mom Now That I Need Her?* With this book, I have never had to buy pancake or biscuit batter (I make my own from scratch, using organic ingredients), I can always figure out something great to do with a thawed chicken breast using the things I already have in my cupboard, I can whip up a satisfying GMO-free dessert any time, and I never arrive at a potluck without something impressive. In addition, this book has tips on car and bike maintenance, first aid, and laundry and clothing repair. There is no need, nor has there ever been a need, to buy spice/seasoning envelopes or batter mixes (which are often high in sodium and unnecessary preservatives and unnatural flavors), or (God help us) frozen entrees (although they can be an occasional treat for a tired single mom. Keep in mind that there is no judgment here—just strategies for a better, happier, healthier way to be).

My kitchen is stocked with the components either to make things from scratch and/or to make vegetables more interesting: Flour, baking soda and powder, powdered chocolate, spices, garlic (I get organic minced garlic in a jar—that way I know it will last even if I don't use it soon after I purchase it), beans, low sodium canned tomatoes (in glass jars), canned pineapple, frozen peas and corn, frozen bread, frozen butter, balsamic vinegar, rice vinegar, olive oil, Dijon mustard, various condiments and spices, etc. The only thing I purchase at the store is perishables, and I make sure I use them up on Saturday (my shopping day is Sunday), or at least take an inventory of what's left and make sure not to buy something I already have. I try to get whatever organic vegetables in season are available at my grocery store, and will sometimes get local non-organic veggies in season if they're not in the Dirty Dozen.

I am also a big fan of local foraging. If you live in a rural area like I do, you may have tons of free food just growing out of the ground or swimming in the streams! In my neck of the woods, I catch all my own of salmon, trout, and halibut (enough to last me a year at the close of the season) and either fillet, vacuum seal and freeze it; smoke it; or can it. I forage for currants and high-bush cranberries and make my own juice and can it on the stove (about three gallons every year, which costs me about ten dollars in gas for the stove and new lids for my bell jars—Compare that to the $100.00 or more that juice would cost as the store). I also gather and freeze my own raspberries and blueberries for smoothies, pancakes, pastries, sorbet, pies, jellies, and juices. I make ketchup out of rose hips. In the spring, I harvest fiddlehead ferns and serve them on the side of my last few fillets of salmon before the next fishing season. I'm too scared to do mushrooms, although I understand that there are several edible types in the woods near my house.

Each year, I try to grow at least two things that grow well in my zone (the yard belongs to my dog, so I grow things in flower boxes), and my neighbors grow other things, and we barter and trade. I try to make things about what I can find locally and for cheap rather than getting an idea and paying money for what's out of season. I also have one little chive plant growing in my window. Every time I have baked potatoes and want chives, I say to that plant, "You're paying for yourself again!" A package of fresh organic chives at the store is about three dollars, the amount I paid for the plant in the first place. I have baked potatoes at least once a month, but haven't bought chives in three years.

Yes, I am a bit of a granola and that just might not be your style. But if you live in a place where you have the opportunity to live off the land, it is a great and healthy hobby for you to get into! An extra bonus: Men really like to go fishing. I have heard that women who fish are "sexy." That might work out to your advantage.

When your baby is old enough to start eating food, having a well-stocked kitchen will save you money. A jar of organic baby food can be expensive. And no matter how expensive baby food is, one very important question is this: Would *you* eat it? Then again, would you eat crushed cooked peas, soft green beans, fresh avocado, smashed banana, or steamed butternut squash? And how much does it cost to put a few peas in a baby food grinder? And whatever is not eaten doesn't have to go to waste. It's not gross, so *you* can eat it! I had a friend who would use her baby's smashed peas to make the best tasting samosas.

Do make sure that what you make for your baby is from fresh sources and cooked by you, as canned green beans and other canned veggies have high sodium (anything more than 30 grams of sodium for a 16 oz. can is too much). Canned baby food is preferable to giving your baby high amounts of sodium.

Get Moderate Exercise
Regardless of how healthy or active you are or aren't, you need regular exercise, and exercise doesn't have to be strenuous to be beneficial to your physical and mental health. Although mild, moderate exercise probably won't help you lose several pounds, that's not what you're aiming for at this moment. What you need to do both now and after the baby is born is to simply get outside, get out into the world, and keep moving.

If you have the time and money to do a prenatal yoga, swimming, or other exercise class, that's great—embrace that opportunity. If not, remember that the world is your gym and it's free. Take walks, go to the beach, go for a bike ride… even walking the mall is better than sitting. If you like a structured workout, there are many prenatal workouts available for free on youtube, or accessible on your streaming device, and of course you can always find second-hand workout DVDs. If all you have time for in a day is a short walk, don't get discouraged and stop. To walk for as few as ten minutes and to stretch for one minute is much better than to do nothing.

Another suggestion: make it easy on yourself to grab a short burst of exercise here and there. Have a Pilates ball in your living room (also makes a good, unobtrusive, extra chair), and exercise bands in your bedroom. If you steal an opportunity to move here and there, your daily efforts may not equal that of a total workout, but your body will be more ready to cooperate when the time comes to *really* exercise.

Practice Meditation, Prayer, or Positive Affirmations
As you may already know, your inner environment is a fundamental component in preventing postpartum depression. If you effectively learn to train your mind to be calm, focused, and positive, you will be able to embrace small opportunities throughout the day to exercise preventative maintenance, and it will be generally easier to bring your energy up after a challenge or disappointment.

If meditation has always seemed too boring to you, now is the time to let those old sentiments die. After the surge in popularity of the movie *What the Bleep do We Know,* many people learned that when a holy monk concentrates his loving and peaceful energy on a glass of water, the water reacts in a positive way to his energy. The human body is approximately 75 percent water. We can actually *change* ourselves through positive thinking, and we can maximize these changes through meditation, prayer, and positive affirmations.

Meditation, like prayer, is simply intense focused thought with a purpose. Very often, people are drawn to meditation when they are looking for a practical way to decrease their anxiety, gain better control over their lives, or to simply glean more joy out of their existence. Methods of meditation vary widely: for example, in Zen meditation, one is not supposed to focus on anything other than simply "being," whereas in Intentional Meditation, one is to clear the mind of any self-undermining thoughts and visualize a positive outcome of their desires for money, love, peace, happiness, etc. These are only two examples from literally thousands of meditation styles that have proven to positively alter the lives of the practitioners.

While you are still pregnant, make a commitment to learn about what works well for you, fine-tune your regimen, and enter into a regular meditative practice to train your mind to 1) focus on happiness, 2) turn towards positive thoughts and expectations, and 3) bounce back to positive thinking after a challenge or a disappointment. It is extremely important to master these skills right now and continue to practice them after the baby comes.

◆ ◆ ◆

Guard Your Post
Although pregnancy might sometimes make you feel like you are merely a host of an alien life form, rest assured that your body is your sacred personal sanctuary. You must do whatever it takes to protect and care for it.

Remember that any help that anyone gives you, be it money, advice, or information should be completely and absolutely unconditional. People who refuse to help you unless you follow a specific path are not helping you; they are manipulating or bribing you. There is a cosmic spiritual plan for you, and you can only follow that plan if you listen to your own heart.

And speaking of your own heart, protect it, strengthen it, and learn to trust it. Know the strength of your heart and mind depend partially on the way you care for your body—they are connected. Toxins and poisons will compromise your ability to be strong. Wash them away with good nutrition, and keep your mind clear and focused on positive things. Know for certain that you have all that you need to succeed and prosper in this life.

It is time to stand strong and guard your post. Do not let yourself be manipulated by any outside forces. Always remember that your heart, your life, your body, and your decisions are precious, and that you are the guardian of these precious things.

Chapter Three

Life Starts Now! Groom Yourself for Greatness

For some, the question "What are you going to do with your life" may bring about a post-traumatic stress reaction to memories of familial disapproval regarding tattoos or prom dates, and for others it might even be the harbinger of a nerve-wracking interview that is soon to come. However, in this context, the question of your life plans should cause you no stress because you are going to answer not to disappointed relatives, judgmental friends, or me. This time, not only are you going to answer only to yourself, but you are also going to be given the tools to make your dreams come true.

For the moment, forget your preconceived notions of what is realistic for your situation. If you allow yourself or others to put restrictions on your life, you will not reach your true full potential. If you accept the fact that progress will be slow, if you have the perseverance to take "baby steps" (no pun intended) towards attaining your goals, and if you accept that success does not happen overnight, the sky's the limit for what you will achieve in your life.

Before we get into our life-planning exercises, take a deep breath, slow your mind and body down, and meditate on the following statements:

> **A slow and steady pace wins the race.**
>
> **You are a strong, sturdy ox that is going to haul your load across this prairie one sure-footed step at a time.**
>
> **Eat the elephant one bite at a time.** (Okay—that one's kind of gross, but you get the point)

If you discipline yourself now to accept a slow, steady pace for your progress, this will prevent you from getting overwhelmed with the future. In this chapter, you will be called upon to embrace your long-term goals for success, and to identify short-term goals in each of these categories:

>   Finances
>   Career/ Educational
>   Personal Fulfillment
>   Parenthood

After your goals are identified, we are going to examine what you feel reaching these goals will do for you and plan your course of action.

This is going to be a lot of fun, so let's get started!

Forget About Limits! Identify your Long-Term Goals.
I am going to ask you to make a very personal piece of art that represents your wildest dreams for success. Even if you don't consider yourself a creative person, this piece of art, however simple or ornate, is going to be your inspiration to keep moving forward even when you feel you no longer have the strength. Don't worry about superficiality, materialism, or realism. We are going to acknowledge, embrace, and respect your fantasies.

Note: Those of you who have seen the documentary *The Secret* may know if this piece as a "Vision Board." I must clarify that the first writing of this book came out before *The Secret* was released, so no, I didn't "steal" the idea from them, thank you. They stole it from *me* (I'm kidding, of course. Nobody stole anything: I was first introduced to the "Vision Board" idea by one of my elementary school teachers circa 1979. Even at the age of nine, I knew that it was a good idea, and have revisited it at various points in my life).

Collect a bunch of magazines and look through them to find things that represent exactly what you want in life. You might decide to select pictures of material things such as a mansion, a cabin in the woods, a sailboat, a four-carat diamond ring, a Coach purse, a Lexus… and/or you may be more inspired by symbolism, such as a picture of a sunset to represent peace and relaxation, roses to symbolize love, or a diverse group of happy children to represent your commitment to a career in child welfare. Whatever your hopes and dreams for the future are, find images that represent any and all of them.

Image Guidelines
Only Beautiful Images Allowed
Make sure these symbols are things you enjoy looking at. If your dream is to have a cabin in Tahoe and the only image you find is of a cabin that's the wrong size or has a bunch of junk in the yard you don't like looking at, keep searching for the perfect image.

No Negativity

If your dream is to one day be a physician and the only related image you can find is an ill patient on an operating table, pass that image by and find something that brings about no indication of sadness, pain, or negativity.

It's About What This Image Means to You

Don't worry about adherence to traditional symbols. For example, if you are a Christian and a picture of sunbeams and clouds represents your idea of God more accurately and personally than the image of a cross, stick to the clouds and sunbeams. Trust me, God won't hold it against you if you express a little individuality.

Avoid Grounding Your Images Too Far Into Reality

Although these images have to be personal, they also have to be symbolic. For example, if you are head over heels in love with a man named Fred, don't include an image of Fred himself, but instead find an image of what you want in a partner. In the event that you find out that Fred is a jerk, you don't want this discovery to ruin the integrity of your image. If Fred is a skier and this is what attracted you to him, instead collect the image of an anonymous skier catching air in the mountains. If you find that Fred is wrong for you, don't let it prejudice you against this skier, as he is not Fred—he represents attraction, freedom, adventure, and your future. These images are about *your* future, with or without Fred!

Furthermore, focusing this type of attention on a real-life individual with whom you don't have a mutual relationship is called "obsession," and it is neither healthy nor ethical. Yes, there is a fine line: We all had posters of whatever teen idols up on our walls when we were young, and probably in our strange ways, fell in love with them too. But what we're doing here is different: When we were teens, our mantra was something like, "He is so gorgeous, I wish he, or someone like him, could be my boyfriend." What we will be doing with our collages is more like "What I see on this collage IS mine." The only *person* one can truly own is oneself. But feelings, experiences, abundance, materials, happiness... those we are allowed to take and keep for ourselves. There *is* enough to go around.

Make Your Image Collection Well-Rounded

Don't focus all your images on any one aspect of your future. Include images that represent career, finances, home, romance, family (including your baby), friends, creativity, stability, adventure, children, travel, spirituality, pets, good food, or whatever else inspires you. Your life does and will continue to include many components. Don't limit yourself by putting all your eggs in one basket.

After you have collected your images, get some scissors, glue stick, and a small piece of poster board (8" X 11" is recommended for this project). You may also decide to add some matting or to frame your work. Arrange the images in a way you find appealing to the eye, and glue them on to the poster board. If you have enough images and are having fun, make two or three collages, but keep them relatively small, keeping in mind that they are not meant to be displayed as centerpieces in the more public areas of your home. After all, you don't want to invite an analysis or critique of all your fondest hopes and dreams or your skills as an artist. Instead, these collages will be displayed in the more personal places where you will encounter them daily.

Once your collage is finished, decide where it is going to go. You could put it on your refrigerator, by your bed, next to your computer monitor, the outside of your bedroom door, wherever. Make sure your collage is well lit and visible, and that you will encounter these positive images on at least a daily basis. When you hang your collage, take special care not to rip it or ruin it with tape (if it is made of poster board, it will likely survive taping, but if it is made simply of paper, it may not), because you might want this collage to accompany you through a couple of relocations or furniture re-arrangements.

After you have hung your collage, regard it in reverence. This is your future. Tell yourself that this is what you're working towards, and that this is what you'll get. Open yourself up to the many facets of your destiny. Feel the positive energy of your images wash away any feelings of hopelessness, fear, and self doubt. There is no other option but for you to have these things in life. Repeat this exercise daily, but don't treat it like a prayer. You can pray for guidance, inspiration, and signs from above that you're headed in the right direction, but getting the Lexus is up to *you*!

Every once in a while, reevaluate your collage and update it. I have kept many of mine, and I look through them as though they were a scrapbook of my dreams, achievements, and changing values (the ability to keep them in a binder another reason to keep the size consistently small). It is often very rewarding to see what I have achieved, and also to learn why some of what I wanted at one time wasn't meant to come into my life.

As I mentioned before, progress for a single parent is slow: [you may remember the aforementioned meditation] Eat the elephant one bite at a time. This is your elephant. Now we are going to figure out how to eat it one bite at a time.

Short-Term Goals
Several years ago, I encountered an extreme energy slump. Three of the biggest of the short-term goals I had established within the last five years had been attained: I had bought a two-bedroom house with a manageable payment in a wooded setting, I was in the process of getting my master's degree at a prestigious university, and my son was healthy, happy, and thriving. I should have been happy. After all, I had everything I

wanted, but something was off. I couldn't find the inspiration to get any work done— not around the house, not in my writing, not at all. When I was sick in bed for three days with the stomach flu, I had a lot of time to think about this: What do I want *now*?

What I wanted more than anything was to find the love of my life, but the world just wasn't cooperating. After all, finding the love of your life involves the cooperation of another human being, as well as your being at the right place at the right time. For finding love, destiny was not entirely in my own hands.

Over the last five years, I had put energy into finding my soul mate. I had gotten myself into physical shape, invested in my wardrobe, my appearance, and my health, had let my friends know that I was open to blind dates, and practically every child-free night I had was spent at the clubs, at the parties, at the restaurants, on the trails, on the rivers, or skimming the photo ads on Match.com. Sure, I'd had some dates, made some friends, and had some interesting experiences, but still I remained without a partner. And I was so focused on attaining the right partner that each of my failures, even if I learned a lesson or made a friend, was a major disappointment and was difficult to put into perspective. I was working hard and getting nowhere. A few times during my bed-ridden stomach flu delirium I sat bolt upright in bed and sobbed, "Why, why, why am I alone, alone, alone?" The pain, the vomiting, and the sadness—it was not fun.

But then I realized what it was that was really bothering me. I had forgotten to re-evaluate my next step in working towards fulfilling my dreams. As mentioned before, I was working hard and getting nowhere, and that's because I was too focused on attaining the goal of companionship, which I could not hold myself accountable to attain. I needed to find something else, something concretely attainable within one or two years, to inspire me to go on. I asked myself, "What is it that would make me happy? What am I going to work towards? What could I possibly get in the next one or two years that would reward me and significantly change my life for the better?"

Did I want a new car? Heck no! Mine was paid for, and in Alaska they just get thrashed anyway. Did I want jewelry? Nah. If you wear anything too big around here, people just assume it's fake anyway. Did I want to travel? Didn't think so. The last time I went overseas I got Salmonella and spent a week in a Czech hospital. It looked as though there was nothing on earth that could possibly make me happy.

And then it came to me: An image from my childhood. I saw myself as a little girl riding a Palomino in an open field on a bluebird sunny day. I felt happy and free. It looked as though I wanted a horse!

But did I want the responsibility of owning a horse? They're really hard to take care of, and one needs either to live on a large piece of property or to have the horse boarded. Was I ready for all that? And although I had some very satisfying horse-riding experiences as a child, the three times in my adulthood that I had ridden had been… well…

awkward and painful. But the image kept coming to me, and the feeling of freedom and happiness that followed these thoughts was undeniable.

I decided to go on the Internet to do some research. I found an equestrian tour in Ireland in which a group of single people ride across the countryside for four days, staying in castles all the while, and end their trip at a famous Valentine's Day Bachelor Auction with an escort provided by the host country.

Wow! This sounded like the vacation of a lifetime, and with the right planning, it could certainly be done!

So there I had it: I had found my inspiration. My first step was to get horse riding lessons. Approximately a year from the date of my epiphany, I would be riding across the Irish countryside and staying in castles. If riding a horse for several days proved to be as rewarding as I had anticipated, my goal within the next year would be to modify my lifestyle to include horse ownership.

Within days I had found a picture of my dream horse, named it, and stuck it on my fridge. For the following two weeks, I was so excited about my new goal that the priority of finding my soul mate was moved down a few notches. If a man had managed to steal my heart within the next year, he'd surely have to be something special in order to change my mind about taking that Valentine's Day horse-riding trip (not to mention he'd have to reimburse me for my deposit)! Having a personal self-fulfillment goal took the pressure off me to put all my energy into finding love.

With your circumstances right now, the thought of riding a horse through Ireland might seem superficial, impractical, selfish, and unrealistic. After all, in the next year you are going to have a baby. There's a possibility that at this moment you don't have a savings account, insurance, a satisfying job, or even a decent place to live. If that's the case, maybe you'll gain inspiration from the fact that six years ago I didn't have any of those things either.

And at this time in my life, I go out at least once a year and do something *amazing*. I have done some things that require that I sought a week or so of childcare from my mom (equestrian trips, for example), and I have greatly appreciated having that option, and I know that not everyone who is reading this book will. But I have done things with my son in tow as well—I have just had to take the "adventure" quotient down a notch or two, and do something that didn't depend on a tight schedule and would make us both happy (beaches, train trips, road trips, resorts, cruises, visiting far-flung friends and relatives at their houses, etc.). As your child grows, he or she will be able to handle, and will be enthusiastic about more.

The secret to getting what you want out of life is to set attainable short-term goals in various areas of your life and to work unilaterally towards attaining them through positive thinking and action. When one goal is attained, it needs to be replaced in order to keep you inspired, and to prevent you from becoming frustrated in the event that the completion of a goal in another area seems to elude you.

Here are some examples of simple goals that can be attained within the time frame of one year:

1. **Financial Goals**

    I want to decrease or eliminate my debt.

    I want to liquidate everything in my household that I no longer want or need and put the money into savings.

    I want to save at least ten percent of every paycheck for a year.

    I want to establish credit without carrying a balance.

    I want to get all my baby gear second-hand

2. **Career/ Education Goals**

    I want to take a six-month class in massage therapy and build a clientele of at least five people.

    I want to take six credits/ units (two classes) towards getting my associate /bachelor's degree/ master's degree.

    I want to get a job/ better job.

    I want to supplement my income by selling my crafts on Etsy.com

3. **Personal Fulfillment Goals**

    I want to walk at least a mile three times a week

    I want to learn to snorkel.

    I want to take a digital photography class.

    I want to wake up early enough to fix my hair every day.

    I want to meet at least one new person every week.

4. **Parenting Goals**

    I want to improve on my parents' upbringing of me.

    I want to keep fast food and sodas out of my child's diet.

    I want to take my child to the park (to church, to a restaurant, swimming) every Saturday.

    I want to feed my child only natural meats and organic fruits and vegetables.

Now let's establish one goal in each category that you hope to attain within the next year. If you plan to set a lofty goal in one category (ex: I want to establish a personal shopping business), try to make your goals in the remaining categories a little less challenging (I want to save money and get exercise by washing my car in the driveway rather than taking it to the car wash).

A good way to keep your goals organized is to take a dry-erase board and post it somewhere in your house (inside the kitchen cabinet is a good, private place to track your progress). Write down your goal in each category and a due date for completion. When a goal is reached, erase it from the board and replace it with another, and re-set the due date. If the goal is attained in less than a year, think about upping the ante next time. And finally, make sure your goals are truly inspiring and are things you are enthusiastic about. *Don't establish goals to please anyone but yourself.*

Guidelines for Establishing Your Initial Goals
Take Baby Steps.
Start small. Keep in mind that the next year is going to be a difficult one with your sudden change in lifestyle. Keep it simple at first—don't put pressure on yourself to do too much, or your goals will become overly burdensome and will take on a negative flavor.

Consider your Current Circumstances Before you set a Goal.
Pregnancy and motherhood can make attaining certain goals impossible. If fitness is important to you, don't require yourself to lose twenty pounds in the next year. Instead, strive to do a pregnancy-safe, low-impact workout twice a week, and re-establish this goal to include the weight-loss addendum and re-set your yearlong time line six weeks after the baby is born.

Think Your Goals Through Carefully.
Yes, you may really, really want a dog, and having a walking companion may help you keep your fitness goal. But dogs can be hard to manage (especially in an urban setting), and once you have the huge responsibility of a baby, you may find that the dog was too much for you, and in setting this goal you may have earned yourself enough responsibility to make anyone crazy (many dogs being rehomed on sites like Craigslist need new homes because the owner is having/had a baby and the dog is too much for them). If you do indeed have an ideal situation and can find the right dog for your lifestyle and limitations, then press forward—but don't act in haste.

Apply this logic to anything that can put pressure on you if you are not able to tend to it regularly: New car with a car payment, a class you must continue to take after the baby is born or else you fail the class and lose your tuition… you get the point. Be excited about your future, but not overzealous.

Identify Only One Goal in Each Category.
Your progress in life does not have to be limited to the goals you set, but if you set too many goals, you will overwhelm yourself. If your personal fulfillment goal was to write

a play, but your friend has taught you how to knit, establish a knitting-related goal after you have finished writing the play. If you find that you excel in knitting and do so without encouragement, you may not need to establish a knitting goal at all, or you may decide that to knit and sell five sweaters is a career and education goal rather than a personal fulfillment goal. Goals are set so we can challenge ourselves. As far as the play in concerned, you've given yourself a year to get it done. Concentrate your efforts on attaining one goal in each category at a time.

Have Your Replacement Goals Ready.
When you find yourself on the brink of accomplishment with a goal, think about what your next goal in that category should be.

Don't jump the gun.
Don't focus your energy on attaining your next goal until you have fulfilled AND evaluated the success and rewards of the last goal completed. If you have a bunch of loose ends that need to be tied up, working towards your goals will seem more like a chore than a fulfilling experience.

Time to Write Your Goals
So now it's your turn! Give it some thought, and identify one goal in each category. Don't set your goals or your dates of completion in stone until you have your dry-erase board.

Coming Up With Your Plan
I met Irene many years ago (in this edition, it should be noted that when I met her, smartphones were not yet a "thing"). She was single, pregnant, twenty-three years old, and worked forty hours a week for minimum wage at a coffee shop. She let me know that for a few years she had entertained the idea of starting a personal shopping business, and she was positioning herself to put her plans into action. Although she had no formal education past high school, she seemed mature, enthusiastic, and smart. I decided to see how well she had planned her new career by interviewing her:

> M: Why do you feel that you are suited to be a personal shopper?
> I: *I love to shop. Whether it's for myself, my friends, family, whatever. And people recognize that I have good taste, and I'm already kind of doing it. People are always asking me what perfume I'm wearing. I tell them I'm wearing Eau De Hadrien by Annick Goutal. When they find out how much it costs, they wonder how someone like me can afford it. But I get it on e-bay. I have it stockpiled. I tell people I can get it for ten dollars less than*

retail, sell it to them, and I've already made an incredible profit. For me, personal shopping is a fun and lucrative hobby!

M: What kind of equipment do you think you are going to need in order to expand your hobby into a business?

I: *I already have most of the things I need.*

M: Give me a list of all of those things you need. Whether you have them or not, I want to know what they are.

I: *I need a computer equipped with a program to make business cards, advertising materials, receipts, and possibly a bookkeeping program, but for now I'm just going to keep close track of all my expenses. I will also need Internet access, a reliable car, a hand truck for heavy things, E-bay and Paypal accounts, a really good stroller with lots of storage so I can work after the baby comes, comfortable shoes, a clipboard, a logo, lots of paper, wrapping materials, and a cellular phone.*

M: How do you plan to build your clientele past your perfume fans?

I: *I'm going to approach all my busiest friends and contacts long before holiday season, distribute fliers in office buildings and on notice boards, and introduce myself and my business at the next Chamber of Commerce meeting. Of course I should also make an effort to always dress impeccably when I'm in public, as this is a form of advertising as well. I want to show my clientele that I know where to get the right things, and it's the upscale clientele that I am going to cater to.*

M: Will shopping for other people really be worth your time? You will be on your feet a lot.

I: *I do think it will be worth my time. So many people don't like to shop, and I do. I know where to get the stuff, I know where to get the deals, and I like to do it. If I need to sit down, there are always benches at the mall. I can take a break. And besides, catalogues charge five dollars to wrap a gift. I can charge five dollars for wrapping gifts, maybe even more if the gift is huge or if my client wants a special presentation.   I can charge for delivery—another five dollars! I can charge an extra ten for a rush delivery, within a couple of days. I can charge five dollars an item to return a gift, maybe even ten if my client wants me to return a gift on the day after Christmas.*

M: How are you going to phase your business into your life?

I: *At first, I am going to work only in my spare time. I am going to have my business license, prices, and paperwork established by October. I am going to start marketing for the holiday season right after Halloween, and*

I am going to do all my business after work and on weekends. I figure I'll get at least some business for Christmas and Chanukah, and I'll include in my advertising that I offer the service of returning unwanted holiday gifts for a fee. After the holiday season, I will evaluate what seemed to work well, and what did not while I keep my current job. I will keep accurate records of my clientele: Addresses, family members' names and ages, types of gifts requested, etc. By Valentine's Day, I'll be ready for my next marketing push. I will contact my clients through a direct mailing, and once again I will distribute fliers. After Valentine's Day, I will do another advertising push to remind people that I am available to buy gifts for birthdays and anniversaries. As other holidays approach, I will be sure to advertise my business in the same way.

M: What are you going to do if you have purchased an item (or several items) that your customer does not want and will not pay for, and cannot be returned?

I: *In most cases I'll be getting the money up-front, and I'll let my customers know that they need to provide me with an accurate description of what they want, or if they leave the item up to my discretion and give me a price range, I will do my very best to please them. But if I do get stuck with something I can't personally return, I'll list the item on e-bay. I will keep my cool with this customer and ask if there's anything I can do to amend the problem, because this is good business practice, but I will reconsider whether I want to make this person's business a priority in the future.*

M: How and when are you going to evaluate your progress and see if this is really a business you want to pursue as a career?

I: *A year after I have started with my personal shopping business, when I get my materials ready for taxes, I am going to look at how much I spent on advertising, how much I earned, and how much time I spent shopping. Based on what I learn, I will decide whether I want to pursue this business as a career, a part-time job, something I want to continue with on a light level until a later date, or abandon it altogether.*

M: If you abandon your personal shopping business, how are you going to make the best of this situation?

I: *I will try to sell my business—but that's not going to happen.*

Three years later, Irene was doing quite well with her business. She kept her full-time coffee shop job for a year after she started her personal shopping business (minus six weeks she took off after her daughter was born), but then decided to pursue personal shopping as her career and abandon her coffee shop job. Although some seasons for Irene were extremely busy and some were very slow, at last check-in (several years ago now) she was making much more money than she was while working full-time at the coffee shop, and her business evolved to encompass running errands for elderly people or busy career couples.

Irene also took her daughter along with her while she shopped. She admitted that the cost-effectiveness of her time was compromised by having her daughter along for the ride, but she saved so much money on child care that she was able to both do what she liked to do, and get out of the house to get exercise and have contact with people and the outside world.

As you can see, Irene had a good plan, and she made it work. Let's take a look at some other amazing feats that were performed within the time frame of one year:

A little over a year ago, I met a young woman who was off to take some stained glass classes, which was something she had wanted to do for a long time. A year later, this young woman was invited to hang her work at a fine restaurant that features the work of a different artist every month. Not only did she sell sixteen of the twenty pieces she hung at the restaurant, but she was also commissioned to make a permanent custom sign for the hosting restaurant for a price that made everyone happy. A year before she had been taking classes. Now she was a professional artist.

At the beginning of her pregnancy, Lori was at a loss for what she wanted to do as a career. After contemplating her hopes, dreams, time limitations, and income requirements, she decided that she wanted to be a massage therapist. She took a course that lasted six months, studied hard and paid attention in class, and was on her way to a new career before her daughter was born. Before she landed her first job at a day spa, Lori gave massages to all of her friends at a discount, earning a few very solid customers for life. After putting in a few months (and earning a few loyal patrons) at the day spa, she was hired on part-time at a chiropractor's office, and then was hired for part-time work at a naturopath's office. Within a year, this woman went from having no job at all to having a great career.

Soon after Adriana's son was born, she was feeling confined. She knew she needed to exercise and socialize in order to prevent herself from falling into a funk, but she couldn't figure out what to do. She was a great Salsa dancer, but there was no place in her small town for her to go dancing, and nobody for her to dance with. She discussed her situation with the owner of her local coffee shop, and they came to the agreement that Adriana could teach dancing at the coffee shop one night a week.

The would-be dancers were few and far between for the first few lessons, but after about a month, the news of this new social opportunity spread, as did the crowd. When

Adriana felt that she had secured enough converts, she started charging five dollars a lesson from each participant.

In well under a year, Adriana was very happy with how her life was going. She had made many friends, had created several dance partners, had gone on a few dates, and was earning about fifty dollars a week just having fun. With the new dance craze that was sweeping her town, the local dance club took a break from their country music repertoire, started playing salsa music one night a week, and hired Adriana to advise them on their music selection. In addition, Adriana and her best dance partners started performing at elementary school assemblies, local fairs, and other events. There was no shortage of students, and Adriana raised her prices and scheduled lessons at the local dance studio, the dance club, and at the coffee shop. Within the year, Adriana went from being lonely and somewhat out of shape to having extra money along with a full social calendar..

Martie had only had one job in her life when her husband left her with one child and one on the way. Despite Welfare, Martie had only enough money to pay her bills and put food on the table. She received only a small amount of child support because the state took most of it to pay back the Welfare she had been getting, and Martie felt like she was going nowhere. She didn't have the skills to get a job good enough to warrant her paying for child care, so she needed to find something that she could do from home.

She researched several work-at-home opportunities, but realized that in order to make it with most of those opportunities, one would have to have advanced sales skills, and living on a shoestring herself, Martie did not feel right about selling a product that her customer didn't really need.

After a few weeks of searching, Martie learned of a company that sold earth-friendly health, beauty, hygiene, and cleaning products. Living in an area where most people have septic systems rather than public sewer service, Martie knew that most of her neighbors would benefit from these products, so she enrolled in the work-at-home sales program.

Martie's sales were slow at first. After three months she didn't want to stop selling, but she didn't think that she would ever make enough money to make a living selling her products. Soon thereafter, there was an outbreak of lice at her local elementary school. It just so happened that a non-toxic product for getting rid of lice was a shampoo offered by Martie's company. Martie took the opportunity to pitch her products at the PTA meeting and distributed fliers for the students to take home with them.

This meeting was the big turning point for Martie. Within a week she was doing a presentation to over one hundred parents in the multi-purpose room of the elementary school. That was the month she stopped qualifying for welfare, but Martie didn't care—she was making five thousand dollars a month.

True, the abovementioned women were organized, motivated, and the universe happened to be cooperating with their efforts at the times that they needed positive change.

Right now, on the brink of your own life change, you have a lot on your plate, so to speak. Remember to set only goals that you are comfortable with, but if you are comfortable with making a significant change in your life, you know exactly what to do.

In addition to taking these important steps in making your life all you want it to be, give yourself a pat on the back for almost fulfilling one very important life goal shared by many people in the world: parenthood. Congratulations! Your goal of parenthood is soon to be attained. You are going to be a mother! Have you given much thought to the fact that some very enthusiastic potential parents will never have a child? For some people, having a child is impossible. For you, it is *imminent*. And if you are committed to being the best parent you can be, nobody will be able to stand in your way of growing your child into an extremely kind, ethical, and decent person. This is one of the most important things in your life that you will do. It is true that many people, maybe even you included, feel that your situation is not ideal. When I was pregnant, I was frightened at the thought of what my life as a single parent would be like. But if I knew then what I know now, I would have been thrilled, and I hope to give you some of the enthusiasm and confidence that I didn't have. As I've said before and will say again, it will be worth all the work. You've just got to keep loving this life that you have and keep moving forward.

Chapter Four

The Truth about Daddies

Those of you who have read other pregnancy preparation manuals have most likely noticed that many books supposedly written to *help* pregnant women devote a lot of ink and paper to stressing the importance of a partner's role in a woman's pregnancy, as well as placing acute emphasis on the value of the paternal role in a child's life. Although most statements concerning "daddy" are obviously thrown in to include the father in what is truly mommy's problem/physical responsibility, some sources even go so far as to cite "studies" (based solely on the popular opinion of those polled) indicating that children without fathers were more likely to end up developmentally slow, emotionally disturbed, or in jail. Some sources even insist that male children who don't have father figures are more likely to "turn out gay" because they don't have anyone to "show them how to be a man." Can you see the fear in such statements? Ask yourself this: What are they so afraid of? Are they afraid that society is going to collapse if women realize that they can act independently of men? And don't they think there are better things to worry about than who our children are going to be sexually attracted to many years into the future? It just so happens that my son is a charming, creative, and ethical genius, but I would have loved him just the same if he hadn't been. He didn't turn out gay, but I wasn't worried about it either way. Our children will be who they are. It is not up to us to project our expectations on them.

    The truth is that such doomsday prophecies are simply not true. The characteristic of gender is secondary to the fact that we are all human. The idea that men's and women's talents and inadequacies complement each other in a uniform manner is completely ridiculous. Children need food, shelter, intellectual stimulation (for some, creative stimulation is more important), and love. Although these components can be optimized by two dedicated adults, neither gender has a monopoly on these contributions that help a person thrive. If the propaganda has gotten to you and you feel as though you are going to be an inadequate parent, read *The Courage to Raise Good Men* by Olga Silverstein and Sylvia Rashbaum (see Recommended Reading list at the end of this book). Regardless of your child's gender, this book will help you to see that your feelings of inadequacy were put in place by a culture that wants to keep you in a position of powerlessness. At the brink of becoming a parent, it is time you know the truth and embrace the power that every human being is entitled to.

Despite my knowing that men and women are equally capable of providing what a child needs in order to flourish, I was still irritated with constantly reading and hearing about the importance of "daddy" while I was pregnant. Yes, my situation was not historically typical, nor is yours. Yes, a father is necessary in the biological procedure of creating a child, and it is true that we generally expect them to stick around at least long enough to see their children born. True, a good husband and father is an asset to both a mother and child. But the fact remains that the right partner can be hard to find, and that even the best partners and fathers have their issues, as no woman enters into a partnership without there being an element of compromise.

When I was pregnant, I shared my frustration with a bunch of girlfriends, some of them married with children, some without; some of them pregnant, some of them single. Despite our diversity, we all witnessed the same thing: Most sources give the fathers of unborn children credit for having done a lot more than they've really done. When a woman gets pregnant, who gains weight? Who has no choice but to stop drinking or smoking? Who gets stretch marks and varicose veins? Who risks her life going through labor? Whose hormones go all out of whack? Whose body turns into a leaking milk machine? Although some husbands are sensitive enough to quit bad habits with their wives and girlfriends, the person who experiences pregnancy is *not* "daddy!"

After a long discussion about our physical challenges in motherhood, we looked through some popular pregnancy manuals for examples of "daddy exaltation," and noted that several popular books threw "daddy" a bone on practically every other page.

One friend observed, "Doesn't sound like any of these authors are living in the real world. There seems to be a great bit of denial going on. Like right here, it says, 'have Daddy rub your feet after a long, hard day.' My husband will poke at my foot for fifteen seconds and shove my leg off his lap. Where can *I* find a daddy robot?"

We found one sentence that was so bizarre it was like a disgusting baby-talk tongue twister. It went something like: "Daddy loves baby as much as he loves Mommy, and he'll still think Mommy's sexy with her big belly in her tiny black nightie." That one made *everyone* sick.

My friends' amusement snowballed into an inspired personal criticism of these authors, eventually leading to a venting session about their partners:

"My husband has never once gotten up in the middle of the night to feed Rebecca. Apparently that's my job. She starts to cry, and he kicks me under the covers."

"Maybe you should pump and use a bottle so that you can make him do it and you can get some sleep."

"Oh, I do," she responded. "Everything is ready for him. He pretends he is taking notes just to humor me in the moment, I guess."

"Well, at least he'll stay home with her and babysit during the day. I went out shopping alone for the first time in six months, and Brian called me on my cell phone an hour and a half later telling me to come home because Johnny was crying and he couldn't handle it."

"That's nothing. I've got you all beat. I'm working my life away to put Fred through law school and pay down our debts, and a month ago he put a piano on our credit card and hid it at his friend's house. I just got the bill this week."

Everyone went silent after that. The unfairness of these situations is something many women deal with in silence, other women fear, and some simply accept as the nature of men.

I wasn't sure I wanted the hear this. After all, these were the men of my friendship community. They were my friends. I saw these guys as great fathers and great husbands, and their marriages helped build the foundation for my faith that I might one day find someone perfect for me.

"No, you *have* to hear this," another friend said. "You have to know how lucky you are."

Me? Lucky? Ha! How the heck could anyone think that I was lucky? I was doing everything alone. Nobody was carrying my groceries for me, nobody was accompanying me on doctor visits. When it was discovered that my son had a healthy heart, healthy organs, ten fingers, and ten toes, my only company was the ultrasound technician (she slapped me a high five). The mere thought of someone willingly rubbing my feet filled me with pangs of yearning. Such was not my reality! It took some time and experience before I was certain that it wasn't their reality either. Of the marriages mentioned above, one of them has failed.

Every relationship involves give and take. Often times the giving and taking are out of balance, as will happen when the roles assigned by our culture don't fit the individual's needs or desires. These next three sections are designed to show you that even when someone seems to have it all, there are important things that may be lacking. In some situations the compromise is worth it; in some it is not. In some situations, making a compromise in order to have a partner is not a wise decision at all.

The Reality of Compromise and the Zombie Effect

Shortly after my son was born, I encountered a woman I had met at childbirth classes who was checking groceries at our local supermarket. She was a beautiful woman with blue-green eyes and curly red hair. Her husband, tall, attractive, and outdoorsy, had sat dutifully by her side, holding her hand in solidarity while she shared stories of her pregnancy complications with the class.

"When I first saw you in class and saw that you were alone," she said, "I prayed for you. I thought about you so many times and thought about how hard it must be having a baby on your own. But now I see your mother in here with your son every Sunday, and I just want to let you know that your mother sure does a lot more than my husband does. My little girl is four weeks old, and I resent having to put her in day care so early just to get back to work."

"Does your husband work?" I asked.

She shrugged. "About twenty hours a week, but he doesn't stay home with the baby, even when he could. My job's the one with the benefits, so I work fulltime. Our baby's in day care for forty-five hours a week, and I am so tired. I don't get a moment to myself, ever. And I spend my break time pumping my breasts! I'm so tired, and I'm so mad that nobody told me what this was going to be like."

A year later, before I closed on the purchase of my house, my son and I were shopping at a local superstore. I was excited about having more than one bathroom in my new house and wanted to decorate one of them for my son. I had found some towels I liked, and started picking out a wastepaper basket to match them. As I was putting the wastepaper basket in our shopping cart, I noticed a woman holding the same item in a different color, speculating aloud about how much she liked the color. I agreed. Her partner approached.

"This is perfect for our powder room," she said.

"Put it back," he snapped.

"But we *need* it."

"Nope," he insisted. "Put it back."

He turned and walked away. I glanced in his shopping basket as he passed. I spotted some fishing gear and a couple of action DVDs. I didn't imagine those were as important to her as they were to him.

She sighed, put the wastepaper basket back on the shelf, and jogged after her husband, her head down. I hadn't considered that it might be expensive, but it was pretty stylish. I turned my own wastepaper basket over to behold the price. It was eleven dollars—a more than reasonable price for a wastepaper basket.

The checker at the market and the pair at the superstore reminded me of a relationship that I'd had long before: I had been engaged to a man for three years before I started to realize that when the going gets tough, not everybody gets going. If only one partner in a relationship is carrying the workload or making all of the compromises for the pair, this partner runs a high risk of suffering what I call the "Zombie Effect."

Now, if there's anything I won't do, it's waggle my finger at you over something I don't personally understand. My having suffered the unjustified finger-waggle was the whole reason this book was written in the first place. I assure you, at one time in my life, I too was afflicted with the "Zombie Effect," and I'm certain that there is a reader or two out there who can relate to the following story. If not, I hope that it at least makes me seem a bit more real to you.

Here's the abridged version of how I came to experience the "Zombie Effect" firsthand:

The relationship was great at first. Otherwise, I wouldn't have been wearing my fiancé's ring on my finger. In the beginning, he seemed smart, worldly, attractive, attentive, politically aware, and subscribed to the philosophy that a man was nothing if not a good provider for his family. But what had started out to be a fairy-tale romance had deteriorated to a miserable situation in which I worked fifty hours a week and came home to a dirty house, no food in the refrigerator, and a fiancé who worked no more than ten hours a week who sat reading the paper on the couch. At the time we were living in Barcelona, and by the time I normally got home from work at 9:30 p.m., all of the food markets had closed. Being the type whose health and mood really suffers without food, I would then have no choice but to go out to eat, charging the meal on my credit card (banks were closed as well, and I couldn't get to one while I was at work), normally bringing my fiancé with me both for company and to fend off the guys who would assume that the empty chair across from me was an invitation for company through the typical three-hour Spanish dinner. My fiancé often insisted that he wasn't hungry but would end up ordering something anyway. After all, he wasn't paying for it!

Throughout my time with him, I had gradually grown accustomed to dealing with a lot of his crap. He often criticized my driving, although I had worked as a professional driver and had never had an accident, whereas he had smugly recounted several fender-benders caused by his own carelessness. We never had any money, and somehow he always insisted that it was because *I* couldn't manage money. We taught English at the same school, and our first class started at the same time, but he'd inevitably take so long in the shower that we'd both be late for work. Sure, I could leave without him, if I wanted to get the silent treatment from him all day. He would often complain about our nonexistent sex life, but how is any woman supposed to want to be intimate when she's exhausted and starving? On occasion, we'd go out to one of the local bars, and he'd get upset because I wanted to drink a cola.

"I thought we were going out *drinking*," he'd say. "Lately you haven't been much fun at all!"

On some weekends I would actually *give* him the equivalent of twenty dollars and tell him to go out and have a good time, just so I could have the flat to myself. Yup, I paid him to go away.

We had done a lot of traveling together, and the fact that I had gotten us lost one time had resulted in his never letting me look at a map of where we were. Sometimes I'd want to duck into shops, knowing that it may be decades, if ever, before I'd ever find myself in this town again. If he wasn't in the mood to "stand around" while I looked around a store, he'd continue walking, forcing me to abandon my post in order to chase him down the street, as he was the one with the map and the room key.

"You don't need any of that stuff in there," he'd say, "We need *our* money for *other things*."

Boy, was I well trained! My dignity was in the toilet! I was in denial that something was dreadfully wrong, somehow convinced that my survival depended on him.

Although it would take several more pages to tell the whole story of the slow decline of my self-esteem, one strange detail of my partner's behavior was that he was humiliated by my habit of picking coins up off the street.

"Didn't your father ever teach you not to stoop to pick up a measly penny?" He huffed, "If you accept money that is not handed to you properly, you're of a lower class."

"No," I had replied, "My family thinks that if you don't grab free money because you're afraid of what other people think, you're an idiot."

I continued to collect my pennies (or, in this case, pesetas) until they were spilling out of their containers. Of all the personal characteristics that I had let go over the course of our relationship, this was a trait that was too ingrained and too beneficial for me to sacrifice. So, my money was taking up space? Too bad. As soon as I had enough time to roll my money, as soon as I could get to a bank and exchange these hundreds of coins for currency, I could buy something material, something just for me, and then he'd know that I'm not a fool because I subscribe to the embarrassing habit of collecting pennies.

A few weeks before our year in Spain was over, we went to the beach with some German neighbors of ours and one of them laughingly offered me five hundred pesetas (about five dollars) to jump into the ocean with all my clothes on. It was a hot day, my clothes would dry, and I was there to swim anyway, so I went for it, and was five dollars richer for it too!

A few days later, I found that my pennies were missing. The culprit: my fiancé. His motive: I should know better than to humiliate him by jumping into the water for people who want to "make fools" of us.

Make fools of us? Who was the fool here? One would think that this would have been the clincher, that his actions would fire me up and help me to realize that my very soul had been thrown away with those pennies, and that I would vow not to endure my hunger to assuage his ego because no one comes between a girl and her pennies, but no, that's not what happened. Three weeks later, we went off to Prague for a month, and I paid for the whole thing on my credit card (I must note: At the time it was cheap. But still).

After our year abroad we planned to move back in with our families (his in Los Angeles, mine in Anchorage), save money for a couple of months, and reunite in San Francisco to get married at our Alma Mater. It wasn't until I was back home with my parents that I realized just how hard I had been working to take care of a man (and an unappreciative one at that), and how many sacrifices I'd made for fear of his leaving, when his leaving would have been the biggest blessing of all!

When he was removed from my life, and I was once again free to live, to work, to eat, to sleep normal hours, to look at maps of where I was going, to drink cola to my heart's content, and to manage my own money, I realized that not only was I *not* in love with this man, but I also hadn't been happy for a long time. Furthermore, with the help of my parents, friends, and employers, I also realized that I was a great driver, a dependable employee, and a likeable person.

How had this relationship turned me into such a zombie? The last two years I had spent with him had been fueled by the memory of who he had portrayed himself to be in our first months together. The deterioration in the quality of our relationship had been slow enough to slip past my awareness until my lack of autonomy had simply become the reality that I accepted. Had we not separated for that short time, I might have actually married him—which is a frightening thought!

To this day, I don't doubt that he really did love me in some way, as evidenced by the hundreds of phone calls I received from him for a year after I let him go, but his profession of love was not enough to foster my happiness and support our lives. If he had encouraged me to be my own person throughout our relationship, if he had given me what I needed to develop and thrive, if he had tried to pull his own weight with our workload, and if he *hadn't thrown away my money*, our relationship might have survived the separation.

Luckily for me, I didn't have a child with him. Many women, even if they are aware of their own unhappiness, will stay with the father of their children simply because they've accepted that this is what they've "gotten (themselves) into." A woman in an unhappy relationship with her child's father normally doesn't want to deprive her child of a father, knows the father will not continue to parent the child if he's not forced to do so through a marriage or committed partnership, and will allow the sense of her own identity to fade from her mind—until it ends.

It takes a lot of work and dedication to keep a relationship going, and although any surviving relationship must be functioning on some level, it might not be the level that is perceived by the outside world. Here are some examples of the types of compromises that some partnered women have made. Although some of them are content and even happy with their relationships, their sacrifices might be more than you're willing to make, and there's no doubt that some of the women in these situations have simply become zombies.

A married friend of mine who has two children, one from a prior marriage and one new baby with her current husband, once told me that she had been wanting to move to a better neighborhood for a long time. She didn't feel comfortable with her older son playing out in her unfenced yard, knowing that her neighbors were car thieves and suspecting that they were drug dealers as well. Although they had money in the bank, her husband insisted that they couldn't afford to move. Soon thereafter, he returned from work announcing that he had just wiped out their entire savings (about eight thousand dollars) to buy a new snowmobile. Shortly afterward he got angry with her for buying a comforter with flowers on it.

One acquaintance's husband works full-time during the week, and then takes off on weekends to go fishing with his friends. When she told him that she would like him to stay close to home at least one day a week, so she could get things done without being interrupted by the baby, he said, "You wanted the kid; I gave you the kid. Now let me have my life!"

Many a mother, both married and single, dreams of the luxury of being a stay-at-home mother, all of her basic needs met through the efforts of a hard-working partner. But one highly educated, former working woman I know started to feel confined and isolated in her situation as a stay-at-home mother with a young baby. She suggested that she go back to work part-time so her marketable skills did not become obsolete. Apparently her request was threatening to the control she'd allowed her husband to have over the family's finances and decisions. He told her that if she went back to work, he would divorce her. His famous quote: "You're a mother. You have no business wanting a life outside the home."

I met another stay-at-home mom at the playground who was eager to find a sympathetic ear about her situation.

"Whenever my husband comes home from work and the house is not perfect, he asks what I've been doing all day. Last weekend he was staying home for the day to watch a football game, and I asked it if was okay if I took the day to go shopping while leaving my son at home. I went out for five hours and didn't feel guilty about it at all. I loved having two free hands for once: One for shopping bags, one for coffee! It was great! Anyway, my underwear had been in rags for a long time, and most of it didn't fit anymore. I didn't know what my size was, so the things I had to get took kind of a long time.

"When I got back, the house was filthy. There were dishes in the sink, chips on the floor, and beer cans all over the coffee table. The first thing I did was change my son's diaper. I think he had been wearing the same diaper all day. So, with a smile on my face, thinking that something might sink in, I asked my husband the same thing he had so many times asked me: 'What did you do all day?'

"He stomped off angrily into the bedroom and slammed the door and stayed in there for the rest of the evening, not speaking a word to me until I went to bed and pressed him to talk to me.

"Our conversation went around in circles, centered around the idea that he thought things were going to be 'different.' I asked him if he wanted a divorce, but he said no. I asked him what I could do to make things better, and he'd just shrug. It just went around and around like this. I didn't know what the heck he wanted me to do!

"Well, I figured it out. After he pulled the same thing on me a couple more times, I realized that it happened each time I actually took him up on his offer to stay at home with our son, when he felt called upon to sacrifice his freedom for a couple of hours so I could live my life. If I take advantage of his babysitting, I end up paying for it with diaper rash, a filthy house, and the silent treatment. These days when I have to do something for myself, I hire a babysitter and do it in the middle of the week when he's not home."

An ex co-worker of mine wasn't exactly complaining about her husband when she mentioned his strange views on breastfeeding.

"He insisted that I breastfeed our son, mainly because he felt that boys who aren't breastfed will turn out to be gay. But he didn't want me to do it in front of anybody."

"Why not?"

"He didn't want other men looking at my tits. He said that he was afraid that it would turn people on or gross them out."

"So where did you go when you were in public?"

"I'd go into the bathroom and sit on the toilet. If we were in a busy place, I'd go out and warm up the car, listen to the radio, and do it there. One time he came out and got mad at me because I didn't cover up well enough. I did a lot of pumping so that I'd have some reserves if we needed it, but he thought that was gross, and he didn't want to see me doing it. He also got grossed out when he'd find it in the freezer. He'd make me hide it way in the back. One time he even threw a bunch of it away just because he couldn't stand the thought of it that close to our food. "

Luckily for her, she seemed amused by her husband's strange reactions to her natural bodily functions. I personally wouldn't have been so amused.

It was actually a bachelor friend of mine who expressed concern over the relationship of his female friend.

"Chris asked her husband to watch the baby regularly on Sunday night, *one night a week*, because that was the only night she couldn't find a babysitter or get her parents, her sister, or anyone else to take the baby. He wouldn't do it. Because she's too 'inflexible,' she couldn't get this job at the best restaurant in town, so she's working as a deck hand a few hours during the day, slinging drinks at night, and he's out partying all over town.

"He spent two months on a fishing boat, and I guess his stint is over, because I saw him at a party last night and he was bragging about how he's just going to 'relax' until he goes fishing again next summer. Then Chris's sister and her husband showed up with the baby, and this guy didn't even seem to notice that his own child was in the room. Word on the street is that the baby doesn't even like him. Go figure."

Who is really doing all the work?
Sometimes the woman is the breadwinner in a marriage. This can work out great in the event that the man is adept at (and satisfied with) taking care of the children. But the fact is, some people are good at taking care of children, some are not. Some people are good at holding on to their jobs, and some are not. Some coupled parents aren't good at either task, in which case, one party has no choice but to do both. True, sometimes an individual will go through a string of jobs that they lose or quit due to personality conflicts, bad work atmosphere, a turn in the economy, inadequate training, faulty communication, or other elements beyond their control. However, there are many hard labor jobs available to untrained, uneducated men for the mere trade-off of passing a physical exam and possibly a drug test. These jobs are also now available to women, but often involve heavy lifting, exposure to toxic chemicals, or are physically taxing. And due to the old patriarchal notion that men should be the primary provider in a partnership, these jobs will typically pay a man an average of 30 percent more than they will pay a woman.

Nevertheless, many women who have babies not only take care of the babies, but they take care of their partners as well. As you will soon find out, babies are not at all easy to take care of. It's fulltime work being a mother. For this reason alone, a hint from any man that he is not any good at taking care of babies should be taken seriously. In the event that the woman in a partnership is the primary breadwinner as well as a mother and is with a man who can't seem to hold a job, then she will either have to buck up and shell out the cost of hiring a babysitter, or she'll risk coming home to a baby who's been shaken to death or a toddler who has choked on something he found on the floor while dad wasn't paying attention.

Some marriages fall apart because of a lack of sexual excitement in the relationship during the postpartum months. Although mothers are warned not to try anything too physically taxing, including sex, until she's been given the go-ahead by her midwife or doctor six weeks after giving birth, most mothers will assure you that sex is the furthest thing from a woman's mind when she's exhausted and still sore from having pushed a baby out of her vagina, and that six weeks is not enough time to get her sex drive back. But the "right" to enjoy a woman sexually is still considered by many men to be one aspect of marriage that shouldn't be put on hold. Some will use their wife's lack of interest and refusal to have sex in the first postpartum months as the excuse to look for it outside their partnership.

Furthermore, it's normal for it to take a while for a woman to get her body back to where she feels comfortable with it, and if her partner shows any displeasure at how her body looks and feels in the months after giving birth, that can really flatten a woman's self-esteem.

After giving birth to my son, I was so busy and overworked that the extra pounds just melted off, and I was back down to my pre-pregnancy size in a year without even trying to lose weight. As one whose priorities were not with impressing men (and one who is painfully aware of the fact that a body considered perfect by the prevailing cultural standard does not in any way guarantee a satisfying love life, as evidenced by model and former fellow single pregnant woman Elizabeth Hurley), I hadn't minded the extra pounds, so I didn't see how anyone would find my weight loss enviable. In addition, I had enjoyed the sociological experiment of temporarily having large breasts, concluding that women with large breasts do have more dating options, although rarely are aggressive suitors the most savory characters around. However, I had failed to consider that throughout my postpartum days, I didn't have anybody criticizing my body. The only witnesses to my body had been my infant son and myself, and after having suffered acne for years in my adolescence, the carrying some extra weight part of new motherhood was no big deal to me.

When I would complain to other new mothers that all I'd had to eat in the past two days had been a peanut butter sandwich, my words would rarely garner understanding. Instead I'd get an up-and-down glance, followed by something along the lines of, "I still don't feel sorry for you."

I didn't think it was very nice to withhold sympathy from a starving woman. After all, I was in pain from hunger and exhaustion. But the more I heard other mothers talk about their lives, I realized how many of them are requested to do every bit as much as I do, and sit-ups as well, just to look good to their partners. I have since learned that when some men start up that "You're not the same person I fell in love with" speech, they are all too often throw in that nice tits and flat stomach that were integral in keeping their interest piqued. Some men threaten to leave their wives if they don't return to their pre-pregnancy size, turning new motherhood into a race for survival: Make fitness you priority, or you'll be eliminated, and I'll find someone else to finish this race.

The above scenarios (and these aren't the worst ones) might cause us to ask ourselves a few questions: Why do some men require their partners to work so hard at keeping them happy when there's a new and completely dependent life in the picture? Why do women work so hard at being sexually appealing to men? Do they do the same for us? And why do we women work so hard at keeping a partner who casually threatens to leave us over something as superficial as a flabby post-birth belly or stretch marks?

I'll tell you why: We women are taught to *fear* solitude. Men are groomed to enjoy their freedom, whereas sometimes we women don't even know what to do with it. Often times we are so afraid to be alone that we can't see that life would require less work and provide more opportunity and enjoyment for us in the event that we were to strike out on our own.

As a single woman who has chosen to keep and raise her child, you will not be sacrificing any of your hopes, your dreams, your goals in life, or the way you want to raise your child for the sake of a man. You will not be used as a free babysitter or a stepping-stone to a better opportunity. You will not be taking care of another full-grown person who is perfectly capable of taking care of himself.

Instead you will be called upon to make a real assessment of what's important in your life. Yes, your child is high on your list of priorities, but you don't have to lose sight of what else you want out of life. Yes, your progress in reaching your personal goals will be slowed significantly, especially within the first two years of your child's life. No, you will not have time to do everything, at least not all at the same time. And, yes, you will make sacrifices in order to take good care of a small human being who is indeed dependent on you. However, beyond what is required of you in meeting your needs and that of your child, you will be living life on *your* terms. Be thankful.

The Logistics of Compromise
When my son was small, I had three girlfriends who were also mothers of children close to my son in age. We had a lot of fun together, but we only got a chance to see each other about once a month. Although I was the only single one, the other three women had absentee partners, so in some ways their lifestyles matched those of single mothers. True, they were not *really* single mothers, but when you take a look at their lifestyles, you might see that their sacrifices were the same as, if not greater than those of us who didn't have partners.

Yes, these women did make sacrifices, and they were even some of the luckiest women around, all of them married to decent, loving, dedicated husbands and fathers; but even these women would roll their eyes and tell you in detail about how some of their husbands' choices had temporarily or permanently altered their quality of life. Although these particular men had proven themselves to have many more good qualities than bad ones, you'll see that their wives were every bit as busy as I was (some even busier), and some had lives that were lonelier than mine.

Linda's husband worked in the oil industry and spent every other two weeks drilling for oil in the Arctic Circle. Linda also worked full-time as a massage therapist, an extremely lucrative but physically taxing occupation. They own a very nice house together, and their daughter goes to day care for approximately thirty hours a week. They are the only ones among us who currently had a combined income, and together they made great money, but they had the expenses of a mortgage, childcare, and various other debts. The three of them traveled by air at least once a year to visit his family in Michigan, and Linda's husband had some expensive outdoor hobbies.

Donna's husband had the same two-on, two-off work schedule as Linda's husband. He worked as a State Trooper in a remote Alaskan Village. Donna, who didn't work, was usually calling around, hoping that one of us could find the time to take a class with her at the Native Heritage Center or thinking that we might have time to spend the afternoon shopping, sunning, or taking a hike. Donna and her husband owned a townhouse together, and their child stayed home with his mother. Of the four of us, she had the most free time. Although we all enjoyed her company, Mickie (see below) and I only got a chance to see her at our monthly meetings, and Linda spent an average of one additional afternoon with her each month.

Mickie's husband was studying to get his doctorate, was in his last year of school, and was living in New York City. Mickie worked full-time to support herself, her two year-old daughter, and to put her husband through school. Her husband would eventually have great earning potential, and was happy to take care of his daughter as well, but Mickie had been supporting herself and her husband since they married. Their daughter came along when her husband was about halfway through getting his degree, and they decided that it was not in the best interest of their future for him to stop his schooling. Mickie and her husband had accumulated lots of debt while putting him through school and because of some luxury splurges before she got pregnant. She paid for a one-bedroom apartment for her husband in New York City and had just bought a small two-bedroom condo in Alaska for the three of them to live in when her husband finished his schooling. Of the four women, she has the highest income, but has the least money to spare. She also had the least spare time.

And then there was me. At the time during which I made this comparison, I had no husband or partner, but I did work about thirty hours a week, and I did get a small amount of support. I owned a home, and I did pay more than average for full-time day care despite the fact my child was never in day care more than thirty hours a week (When you find the right daycare, the expense if often worth it). I could also rely on my parents and to take my son two or three days a week all year round, if needed.

Now it's time to compare our situations:

Which family had the highest family income?
1. Linda
2. Mickie
3. Donna
4. Me

Which mother had the most free time?
1. Donna
2. Linda
3. Me
4. Mickie

Which families spent the most on housing and debt?

Linda's and Mickie's families spent more than 50 percent of their incomes on housing and debt.

Donna's family and I spent less than 50 percent of our incomes on housing and debt.

Who had the fewest family members to take care of?
1. I had to support one adult and one child
2. Mickie had to support two adults (one of them a student) and one child
3. Together Linda and her husband supported two adults and one child.
4. Donna's husband had to support two adults and one child.

Who paid the most for housing?
1. Mickie (one condo in Alaska and one apartment in NY)
2. Linda (one expensive house)
3. Me (had bought my house recently)
4. Donna (bought hers three years before when prices were lower)

Based on what you can see here, you may observe that I had created a pretty good balance between work, financial responsibility, and spare time, despite the fact that I was single. Here are some other conclusions you can draw based on the above comparisons.

Some women, despite the fact that they are married…

…Work harder than I do

…Have less money than I have

…Have less free time than I have

…Are lonelier than I am

...Have more people depending on them
...Spend less time with their children than I do
...Have to work despite their husband's income
...Have more financial responsibility than I have

Surprised? Of course you are. Our society would have you believe that a married mother's life is all about minivans, soccer practice, and Jell-O, but what you see here is the truth. For most people, it's a lot of work, no matter how you slice it!

Of all of these women, the one who worked and sacrificed the most was Mickie. She worked a full-time job, supported two households, and put her daughter in day care for about 50 hours a week. She saw her husband for about three weeks every six months, and then had to pay off the cost of flying him up to see her. In a little over a year, her husband would have his doctorate, and he would probably find a job for when he got out of school, but they'd have tens of thousands of dollars of debt to pay off after he graduated.

As a single mother, my heavy workload (if you count my pregnancy) lasted for about two and a half years. By the time Mickie's husband had his doctorate, she had been carrying the full load of supporting everyone for six years, and were living in poverty, despite her husband's title, for another four years. For that time, she had no luxuries, she didn't go out to eat, she slept on an air mattress with her two year-old daughter, and she shopped at Salvation Army. She was working towards her future. Sure, she had friends... once a month.

Yes, working and keeping an eye on your goals is going to be hard, but I hope that the act of peering into these women's lives will help you see that the hard work doesn't go away when a person finds love, and that loneliness might still be present in the event that one does. There may be a couple of years that you are going to have to be like Mickie and aim all your efforts towards your future with confidence that you will cash in on all the benefits at a later date. If finding love and having a husband is an important goal for you, think of the fact that Mickie is working towards having her husband just like you are, the only difference being that Mickie already knows who he is!

When Compromise is Not in Order
Throughout the last few pages, you have seen how some women have had to weigh the benefits and drawbacks of their relationships and make choices as to whether or not their situations were healthy or acceptable. Some of us wouldn't tolerate their situations, and some of us would. And we've seen that even when the sacrifices are worth it, there is still a lot of work. However, there are certain situations that a woman should never tolerate,

and if she does, she's not only putting her own hopes and dreams on the chopping block, but she's also risking the life of her child as well.

In certain situations, the value that society places on the child's having a father figure just becomes ridiculous. Following are a few examples of what a woman should never tolerate, especially in the event that there will be a child involved. If the man who walked out on you (or the man you sent on his way) has any of these characteristics, be glad that he's no longer in your life, and don't let him come back in no matter what he promises.

Emotional Abuse

We have already seen examples of emotional abuse in **The Reality of Compromise**. We saw examples of men who expected their wives to work to the point of exhaustion, men who criticized their women for physical changes beyond their control, men who put their "needs" far ahead of those of their wives and children, and in the case of my ex-fiancé, men who did their best to make their girlfriends lose their self-esteem so they would remain in control. Being with a man like this is in no way preferable to single motherhood. If the father of your child was anything like this, be thankful that he has gone down the road, and don't accept another man like this in your life again, especially while your child remains in your care.

The definition for Emotional Abuse is so broad and the illustrations so numerous that it would take a whole volume of books dedicated to examples in order for one to get the whole picture, and we don't have time or room for that here. To get a more complete definition of emotional abuse, simply do an Internet search on the subject. Often you find that someone has emotionally abused you when you thought they were just giving you tough love, but if you suspect that you have been emotionally abused, you're probably right. The beauty of being an adult is that you can establish limits on bad situations, and that you are free to leave. The same cannot be said for a child. Make no mistake about it: If someone has been emotionally abusive to you, there's nothing to keep him from being abusive to your child.

Physical Abuse

When I was living in Spain, I was vexed by the fact that Spanish culture often excuses a man's violent misbehavior as "passion" rather than calling it what it is: physical abuse. In a very popular movie starring Antonio Banderas called (in America) *Tie Me Up! Tie Me Down!*, a starlet is kidnapped and physically abused by an obsessed stalker who'd had sex with her once in the past. Eventually she submits to his advances (the biggest argument about this movie is whether or not what he does to her can be considered rape), and suddenly, remembering who he is based on his powerful lovemaking, she immediately falls in love with him. To anyone who's been stalked or raped before, that's really "not too cool."

Although, thanks to growing awareness, it happens less frequently these days in our culture, images of abuse have slipped into our media, and sometimes we, the audience, are manipulated into sympathizing with the abuser's having been driven by his passion and love for his victim to act so out of character.

Take for example the movie *Purple Rain*, starring the artist formerly known as Prince, a movie I watched several times in my early teens. In one scene, the protagonist backhands his girlfriend for her decision to join the band of his rival, not a minute after she presents him with the gift of a very expensive guitar! Eventually, they reunite, and she forgives him. It wasn't until I watched this movie in my adulthood that I realized how wrong the protagonist's actions were. In my youth I had seen this movie countless times, and had still perceived Prince to be the hero, justified in beating his girlfriend because in his perception she hadn't been entirely loyal.

Similarly, in the Richard Gere movie *Internal Affairs*, the protagonist smacks his wife, *in public* no less, knocking her down in front of several witnesses, after his oppressors have manipulated him to believe that she's been cheating on him. Later on in the movie, he rescues her from those people who had convinced him that she had cheated on him. What does *she* do? She doesn't put a lot of thought into worrying about what he's done. After all, he did save her in the end. She forgives him.

These movies seem to buy into the philosophy that a woman is a piece of property that a man can slap around when she makes decisions that he doesn't like, that his inability to control himself was understandable, and that eventually, if *she's* the right woman for *him*, then sure enough, she'll forgive him.

Make no mistake about it, we women have been *trained* to tolerate physical abuse when done in the name of jealousy, understood by many to be a by-product of love. If you have ever had a partner who has slapped you, shoved you, backed you into a corner and yelled in your face, blocked the door so you couldn't leave, ripped something out of your hands, prevented you from eating when you were hungry, driven recklessly while you were in the car, jerked the steering wheel out of your hands while you were driving, pulled your hair, locked you out of the bathroom, thrown things at you (regardless of their aim), choked you, or hit you, you have been physically abused. If you have ever been with someone who has hurt your pets, destroyed your property, or helped themselves to private things like you diary, cell phone, or e-mail, then physical abuse was sure to follow. If you've ever had a partner do any of these things to you, there's no doubt that your child would eventually have earned his time in the spotlight as well. Although an occasional spanking for dangerous misbehavior is sometimes an occurrence in the normal upbringing of a child of loving parents, abusers don't know where to draw the line.

If a man who has been a physical abuser commits himself to an ongoing anger management program, you may consider forgiving him, but it is still a very big risk. If you decide to give this guy another chance, agree to see him only in public, and make this probationary period last for two years. This will show you how strong his love is, but I think you would choose to move on regardless.

It is true that *some* children who see their mothers subjected to abuse all their lives use their experience to vow never to do the same to another human being. If that's the case, I ask you this: How would you like to be the chalkboard in that classroom?

If this sounds like anything that happened in your past, be glad it's over, and vow never to accept this in the future, for your sake and for that of your child.

Sexual Misconduct

As with physical abuse, we are trained by our culture to excuse the sexual indiscretions of men. Take for example the movie *The Crucible*, starring Daniel Day Lewis and Winona Ryder (I have chosen to use the movie rather than the Arthur Miller play for this example due to its accessibility). In the movie, the protagonist, a married man, is understood to have seduced a young girl. Having subsequently realized that his actions could be hurtful to his family, his decision possibly aided by his simply having tired of his paramour, he then rejects his young lover, who decides to retaliate with accusations of witchcraft. At the end of the movie, the protagonist and his wife are being burned at the stake. He insists that he is not guilty of having practiced witchcraft, but he doesn't confess to the real reasons of his having angered his accuser either, possibly because he's confident that his confession will not earn him a lesser sentence, although he doesn't seem to consider that it might clear his wife.

After viewing this movie, many people will condemn the bloodthirsty enthusiasm of the young girl who started it all. Granted, she is no saint. But what many fail to consider is that this little "bitch" is in fact a child whose only sin at the beginning of the story was the fact that she was irresistible to a married man. After being seduced, she is well aware that as far as her religion is concerned, she is already damned, incapable of redemption. Frustrated by the limits imposed on her by her strictly religious and judgmental community, she refuses to accept the fact that she has been used and cast aside, and she decides to take a few of her neighbors down to Hell with her. Who can blame her? She's a child. When a child is struck by another child, she will normally strike back. Many people sympathize with the protagonist: "He made a mistake. He's sorry for it. He does everything he can to save his family, and he never practiced witchcraft!" But he took sexual advantage of a young child, ruining *her* life forever. A few friends of mine and I share the opinion that he got exactly what he deserved.

Having worked for many years in outdoor professions, I have come in contact with a lot of men, and I have many male friends. I have found that there are plenty of men in this world (although hard to find) who are perfectly capable of understanding that a woman (or a child) is a human being rather than an object. I know men who are uncomfortable with the idea of pornography, aware of the fact that there are men in this world who would think nothing of raping, abusing, and exploiting the important women in their lives. I have seen unmarried, uncommitted men, even the loud-mouthed types who are always making crude jokes and don't seem to have many options, turn down sexual opportunities that were, in the physical world, completely free of consequence. I have known men who can appreciate and care deeply for several women while only wanting to be intimate with their mates. I have known thirty-five year old men who have absolutely no interest in women fourteen years their junior, let alone those who are barely legal. On the other hand, I have also known men who make excuses for their misbehavior, but these are never the men who end up becoming my friends. When some men assert that no man can sexually control himself, rest assured that this individual cannot speak for all men. He is simply admitting (and refusing to take responsibility for) his own lack of control.

Granted, traditional relationships can be very limiting in their expectations and their rules, and some people maintain happy and healthy relationships that are non-traditional, mainly because there is honesty and mutuality involved in the standard being exercised. The flipside of the sexual misconduct coin is that a marriage or a commitment is not an automatic ownership contract over another person's genitals (although many assume either correctly or incorrectly that their own marriage is exactly that). I know of many happy couples who have sexually strayed from each other only for the experience to have actually strengthened the foundation of the relationship. Additionally, I know of people whose marriages and partnerships are based on children, finances, and the household, and who love each other and their families very much, but still maintain relationships outside the marriage. In my opinion: To each his or her own. If members of a couple are honest with themselves and each other, they may find this acceptable, but in order for it to be acceptable, it has to be approached with honesty and mutuality: No double standards. What's good for the goose is good for the gander. What would make this a horrific and abusive scenario is if one member of the couple is adhering to a certain standard, believing that this adherence is what was agreed to in the commitment, the other is not, and is not being honest about it.

All things considered, also know for certain that if you have sexually strayed from a relationship, regardless of the circumstances, your genitals are not another person's property. If having done so goes outside the commitment you had with someone, the proper thing for him to do is *not* to beat you, berate you, slander you, or harass you. The proper thing would be for him to break up with you, and set you both free so that you can find something mutual. If this man loves you enough to give you another chance, always remember what's on your record. The likelihood is that the playing field will eventually even up in one way or another. Is your love for him strong enough to forgive as well?

True, many romance movies, as we as our patriarchal culture will often have you believe that cheating is the worst thing that lovers can do to one another, and that there's no "coming back" from the trauma of infidelity. In my experience, when there's real love involved, infidelity and the anger surrounding it can indeed be overcome.

Pedophilia, on the other hand (a sexual attraction to children), is something that, if it can be overcome, is still too much of a risk for any mother to tolerate. If you ever find yourself with a lover who you even suspect might have this problem, close that heart. Cut and run. You owe him nothing. You owe your child protection, and you owe yourself more. If you have evidence that he has harmed someone, *please* find it in your heart to report him to the authorities. I also have a very hard time excusing or understanding any other type of sexual tendency or fetish that involves violence, or that does not involve consenting adult human beings behaving towards each other in a loving way. Some couples enjoy watching pornography, but most women find themselves extremely uncomfortable when the female subjects are engaging in acts that seem painful or disrespectful to their bodies. Every human being has a right to say no to exposure to things that make them feel bad, sad, or confused. Please be strong and uphold high standards for what you are exposed to. Many women, some of them mothers, have settled for sexual misconduct in their partners for fear of being alone, and at the expense of their children and themselves.

My community has a mandatory registry for past convicted sex offenders, which can be accessed by going on-line through the State of Alaska Department of Public Safety web site. Although many dangerous people have never been caught, one cannot argue that anyone who ends up on the sex offender registry is someone who should not be considered for a partner, even in the event that their crime was the simple act of "grabbing a woman's ass" while supposedly too intoxicated to know better. True, there are some people who end up on the registry for, say, an eighteen year old dating a sixteen year old, the father finding out, and taking legal action. But really, there are other fish in the sea. As a mom, you can't take the risk. Sure, someone may find that he is truly a wonderful soul who made a mistake, or was framed, and deserved a chance, but that can be ventured by someone who doesn't have children.

Often times the true nature of these offenders' crimes are euphemized, as in the case of a one-time friend of a co-worker who had admitted to having raped his daughter while drunk. Shocked and frightened by this man's confession, my friend then looked him up on the Sex Offender Web Site to find that his crime was listed as "Attempted Third Degree Sexual Assault of a Minor," illustrating that the prosecutors couldn't get enough evidence to nail him for all that he had done, giving prospective employers, friends, and neighbors the false idea that he "might not have been so bad." Some people have a problem with the registry, stating that having one's picture and address on the web site goes against an individual's right to privacy, and many listings, including that of my coworker's one-time "friend," have been purged because attorneys have successfully argued that those offenders whose crimes occurred before 1984 might not have done their deeds if they had known the public humiliation associated with the web site. In my opinion, a sex offender shouldn't have a right to privacy, an open door to commit their crimes again without the public having been warned. I don't feel that we should commit arson on these peoples' houses or harass them (there is a fine line between self-protection and becoming a villain yourself), but we should definitely be aware and steer clear. It is true that sometimes people slip through the system and are never caught, but if you have access to such a web site in your state, I recommend that you use it in order to know who to be careful of in your community and in your personal relations.

If you have any indication that a man is creepy, regardless of whether or not you have hard evidence, *for God's sake, head for the hills!* You may be wrong, but your life and that of your child depend on your erring on the side of caution. As an adult, you are capable of rejecting men who subscribe to sexual misconduct. Be thankful that there's nobody you have to deal with right now.

Alcohol and Drug Abuse

Many women find themselves in love with men who abuse drugs or alcohol. Sometimes they tolerate and work with their partners to conquer their addictions. But my advice to anyone currently operating without a partner is this: If a prospective partner has failed to gain absolute control over a past problem with drugs or alcohol, don't fall in love with him. It's the only way to assure that you and your child are safe from something that can chemically alter your partner's ability to function.

Sure, he may be a nice guy with a beautiful soul, and he might be capable of great things when he's sober. But if he has a problem and he's not always sober, he can't be held accountable for how he behaves.

Many people can drink alcohol responsibly, and make adjustments to ensure their safety and that of the people around them in the event that they drink too much. Some people use marijuana to treat or ease the suffering of various medical conditions, including depression and Seasonal Affective Disorder, without it altering their ability to distinguish right from wrong. However, an addict who is not in recovery is one who can't say "no" when the situation clearly calls for them to do so. If you already have one life dependent on your good judgment, you don't need this. If you choose to have a partner, you deserve someone who is fully accountable.

A good-hearted alcoholic is still a threat to everyone when he is drunk behind the wheel, and someone who truly loses their concept of who and what they are when they are intoxicated just might mistake your child for a sex object, an enemy, or someone who is capable of taking care of themselves. This situation is too much of a risk. Avoid it at all costs.

Deadbeats
Anyone who refuses to take responsibility for past mistakes, whether their indiscretions involved financial debts, unfulfilled commitments, or "illegitimate" children, has no place in the life of a mother who is working hard to get her life in order and do what's right. Some women will bring men into their lives believing their stories of having been manipulated and trapped by some "bitch," coerced into copulation that resulted in a child he does not accept because he was never in love with its mother. Sure, she might have been awful, but is that the child's fault? And how hard has he worked to try to gain visitation with this child? If the mother is really a witch who only wanted the child as a tool to hang on to him, and if his past is really as squeaky clean as he says it is, regular visitation should be easy to arrange, shouldn't it? Do your best to see all sides of this situation, and don't let yourself be next in line.

And what about those financial problems? Any goods or services rendered that have not been paid for have in fact been stolen, and sometimes thievery is euphemized by this excuse: "I have some debts that I can't pay." Sure, you might have some debts too, but your debts are your own responsibility. Don't let yourself become responsible for anyone else's stolen goods. A good rule of thumb in bringing new men into your life is this: Keep that pocketbook closed. Your responsibilities are more valid than those of some man on the run. Let any man who comes into your life foot the bill for a while. Furthermore, if you start taking care of a man, you'll be giving your own child's money away.

If anyone seems to be "after" a man, regardless of how he tried to explain it away, they are usually after him for a legitimate reason. Don't let anyone hide behind the honesty of your life. If this man is indeed truthful, the facts will surface in due time. But keep your eyes wide open when dealing with someone who has a checkered past. Anyone who seems to be running from a situation is often times running because he's being chased, and people don't often chase just for exercise.

Be smart about your life and that of your child. Never subject your family to a compromise of your safety for the sake of saving yourself from loneliness. In the event that the natural father of your child has the characteristics of an emotional abuser, a physical abuser, a sexual abuser, an addict, or a deadbeat, do yourself and your child a favor and leave his name off the birth certificate, his surname off your child, and his memory in the past. When your child grows to adulthood without ever having been negatively affected by the bad habits of this man, you'll be glad you did.

♦ ♦ ♦

So there you have it: The truth about "daddies" is that they have the potential to be every bit as much, if not *more* work than babies! It is true that love can be a wonderfully satisfying natural high, but just like anything else that makes you high, love can cripple you too. Now that you know the truth, don't subscribe to the idea that things would be rosy if you had a partner. Don't ever crumble under the pressure to have a partner if you're not certain that this is the perfect partner for you, because even if he is, there will be ample sacrifices to make. Don't compromise your very high standards for the company you keep, and don't ever let yourself fall victim to the "Zombie Effect."

On the other hand, if having a partner is important to you, honor that goal. Think about what you want or need, and don't compromise on what you need. Make a list of the characteristics you want in a partner, and know in your heart that these are the characteristics you deserve to have in a mate. The next time a potential partner enters your life, refer to this list, and make sure all of your desired characteristics are addressed. You deserve only the best for yourself and your children.

Chapter Five

A Little Cash Never Hurts!

Although it might be an unpleasant experience, it is time to take a serious look at your financial picture. This may cause you some stress, especially if you are working forty-hour weeks for minimum wage or if you're currently carrying thirty thousand dollars in credit card debt with 22 percent interest. Regardless of what difficulties you might have incurred over these years, if you are truly committed to the project of bringing up your baby (and I know you are), whatever financial challenges you have *can* be worked out.

In the following chapters I will delve more deeply into the specific ways you can acquire funds and cut costs on necessities, but I would like to take these next few paragraphs to help you look at the "big picture." For some reason (I personally blame our culture, but that's just me), many American women have no idea how to manage their money and stay out of financial trouble, which is something you have to learn in order to be a single mom. In addition, our nation's banks and credit card companies have lent irresponsibly to consumers, knowing full well that these consumers had little or no chance to manage the amount of debt they found themselves in. You might already know what to do in order to prepare yourself for the future, especially if you have worked in banking, have taken classes, or have simply learned your skills from the school of life, but just in case you don't, the following paragraphs are full of sound financial advice, and I recommend that you read every paragraph, even if you think it may not apply to you.

If you have an extremely low income and have no debt, you are much better off than someone with a larger income who has a lot of debt. If you have little or no debt, at least you know that the money you earn belongs to you and not Bank of America. Also, you are probably more disciplined than someone with a higher income and can say "no" to yourself when it is necessary. Look into qualifying for WIC (Women, Infants, and Children Program) and Medicaid as well as every other form of assistance available to you, and start saving 10% of each paycheck. If you continue to save 10% of each paycheck, you will eventually have enough of a financial cushion to handle almost any problem that comes your way if you keep your spending under control.

You may eventually want to get *one* credit card so that you can establish credit, but when you have a low income, it is especially crucial that you never charge more than you can pay off in a month. IF you can (and do) pay your credit card off every month, you are beating the banks at their own game. However, if you carry a balance from month to month, even if it's a small one, you are paying for far more money than you ever borrowed.

Credit cards are good things to have for emergencies and once-in-a-lifetime opportunities, and in some cases it is necessary to establish and prove that you have good credit in order to buy a house, but credit balances can get out of control very quickly. Credit card companies are not sufficiently regulated, are out of control, and have a whole slew of nasty tricks up their sleeves: They send you their bill without giving you enough time to pay it (thus accruing late fees and ruining your credit), they hide important facts in the microscopic writing on disclosure forms, they send you notices that your terms will be changed if you don't call them within so many days of receiving the notice (I saw one of mine jump from 4.9 percent to 22 percent), and they'll tack hidden charges on to your account. In addition, some banks have their fingers in some nasty pies: Genocide, irresponsible chemical companies, foreign wars... when you have a card with these companies, your money is supporting these things too. The best way to protect yourself and keep your money karma nice and clean is to have only ONE card from a small, LOCAL bank or lending institution, and pay attention to everything they send you. Credit unions have a more personal relationship with their customers than big banks do, and investing money in your community helps keep your local economy healthy.

If your income is extremely low, sometimes it is better to save in a Piggy Bank than in a financial institution. When I was pregnant, I was denied Medicaid not because my income was too high, but because my savings account was too big. A good friend of mine, who had one hundred per cent physical and financial participation from her boyfriend and had blown all her cash on a brand new car, qualified for Medicaid. Sure, I had a large chunk of money in the bank, but that money had been acquired after years of denying myself luxuries while working in low-paying jobs, and every penny of it (and then some) was spent on doctor bills during my pregnancy, labor, and delivery. By the time my son was born, I hadn't a dime to my name, and had to rely solely on the charity of my parents, extremely lucky to have such an option available to me! Is this fair? No. Is this what the system was put in place for? Of course not. Although the rules for Medicaid have recently changed for the better, we can't see for certain that they will not change again and again, and possibly for the worse. Do your research on the current policy and act accordingly to ensure your survival. Do be honest to a fault when filling out paperwork about how much money you earn and how much money you have in the bank, but what you have lying around the house is nobody's business, especially in the event that what's lying around is a result of your super-human self-control. In the event that you truly have nobody helping you out financially, this is not greed or dishonesty— it is survival. Keep the maximum amount of money allowed to receive aid in the bank, and keep the rest under lock and key at home. In the meantime, do not hesitate to spend money on necessities for you and the baby because strollers and baby gear are of much less interest to others than a pile of money is.

If you do decide to save your money at home, keep it locked and extremely well hidden in a fire-safe box, don't tell anyone (not your mother, not your best friend, not your roommate) where it is or even that you save money at home; and don't even try to do this if your security is compromised by roommates, landlords, irresponsible family members, or nosy guests.

If you have racked up a lot of debt, do not be ashamed. There was a time in history when shame associated with debt was reasonable (when the person who approved your loan was the banker down the street who had known your family for three generations), but these days, people in debt are most often either victims of predatory lenders, or people whose life circumstances changed too quickly for them to financially keep up. If you have a high level or debt but can still manage your payments, what is most important for you to do right now is to diminish or eliminate your debts by any means possible.

If the amount of debt you have is high but manageable (your payments, although you'd rather not have them, don't compromise your ability to feed, house, dress, and transport yourself), the best thing for you to do is to keep your credit rating high by simply pay them down. Sure, some of your friends may be eliminating everything with bankruptcy or debt reduction plans, but they will likely have trouble getting a house or a car within the next few years. In addition, if you own a house, declaring Bankruptcy or entering a debt reduction plan may result in the banks having a lien on your house.

As you probably know, borrowed money is more "expensive" over time due to high interest rates. If you have a large sum of money in a savings account and have a high amount of debt, compare the interest rate on your savings to that of your debt. If your interest rate is higher on your debt than on your savings (which will most likely be the case), it is sometimes better in the long run to sink as much money as you can into your debt and have a smaller savings account. Also, always pay more than your minimum payment on your debts. When you are paying the minimum, you are paying mostly interest and only a tiny bit of principal (the money you actually owe). Credit accounts calculate monthly payments so that if you pay the minimum, it will take you forever to pay off your debt, and they will have garnered much more money through the interest you've paid than you ever borrowed. Again, promise yourself to never be late on credit card payments because a late payment will end up hurting you much more than it will hurt "them."

If you have several credit cards you are paying on, you may want to consider getting a very aggressive debt consolidation loan so you only have one payment to worry about and budget for. If you do this, select the credit card you like the most, keep that one open, and cancel the rest. If you rack up debt upon debt, you will end up in worse shape than if you never got the consolidation loan.

Also keep in mind that debt consolidation loans rarely have low interest rates, but don't let a low interest rate be the reason you don't get one. They are designed to get you out of trouble more quickly than staying with your credit cards. One way to look at it is that if you have low rates on your cards, you will spend the same amount of money paying them off slowly as you will paying off a consolidation loan quickly. Again, see what's available at your local credit union. If you're going to be putting money into something, it might as well be your local economy.

If your debt is clearly too much for you to manage, again, do not be ashamed. The banks who lent your more money than you can ever pay back are fully aware of the fact that they've got you and so many other good people by the "short and curlies." The good news is that you still have options! Depending on your situation, you may opt for a debt relief program, go to credit counseling, or talk to a bankruptcy attorney about filing for bankruptcy (bankruptcy attorneys will often give you a consultation for free). Following are some of the positive and negative aspects of each option at the time of this writing. If you are curious about any of these options, make sure you talk to the appropriate counselor or attorney, as this is just a *very abbreviated* explanation of some of your options, but nonetheless options you may not have been aware of.

Credit Counseling:
Benefits: Credit counselors can lump all of your unsecured debts into one payment with a consistent interest rate. People are far less overwhelmed when they only have one bill to pay, and your credit may remain good throughout the process.

Drawbacks: If your cards have an interest rate lower than that which is offered by the counseling agency (15 percent at this time), your minimum payments will be higher than what you're paying now.

Debt Relief Programs:
Benefits: The amount of money you owe can be decreased *significantly* through negotiations between your creditors and the debt relief counselors. When your payment schedule is satisfied in full (often in three year's time), you can begin to rebuild you credit, and can often achieve good credit once again.

Drawbacks: Your credit will be ruined for the next three years, and that might make things extra tough when you have a new baby. Also, in order for the companies to negotiate your debts, you have to stop paying them, and then you're subject to telephone harassment from your credit card companies until they start to understand that you cannot and will not pay them until you reach a settlement (this can be extremely stressful). It may be much easier to reach a settlement if you have lots of old debt on several credit cards from several companies—if all your debt is from one company or is relatively new, the creditors are less likely to settle with you.

Bankruptcy:
It should be noted that bankruptcy is very complex, and only a bankruptcy attorney can evaluate whether or not it will work for you, and which type of bankruptcy will work best for you. The decision to declare bankruptcy should not be entered into lightly, as it has long-term consequences. However, there are some situations in which it is the only way to address one's financial hardship. Some people claim that the decision to declare bankruptcy was the best decision they had ever made. It is entirely individual.

Benefits: You may be able to get all your debts legally eliminated.

Drawbacks: If you own a house, you may be required to refinance your house in order to pay your debts, which might leave you with a larger house payment than you can afford. You *will* have to go to court, and the thorough examination of your spending habits will be comparable to having a camera up your nose announcing to the world how often it's been picked. Bankruptcy does cost money, as the attorneys need to be paid, and sometimes the creditors get partial payment as well. Although your credit will not begin to repair until seven years have passed, predatory lenders will be alerted to your "debt-free" status as soon as you're through Bankruptcy court *knowing* that you are a "bad gamble," suspecting that you have little or no spending discipline, and hoping they can nail you on late fees, variable interest rates, and hidden charges, as it will be some time before you could declare bankruptcy again. If your house or other assets were protected in your first bankruptcy, they probably wouldn't be in your second.

Unpaid taxes can hurt your future as well. If you have a large amount of taxes that you have defaulted on, the best way to deal with it is to work out a payment plan with the IRS. In some cases (especially if your income has been consistently low), you may owe less than you thought you did, and sometimes a certain amount of your taxes will be forgiven. In other cases, the IRS can drain your bank accounts for the money owed, and you don't want to be stuck with no cash after your baby is born! Ask a CPA ahead of time what she charges to figure out your tax situation. It will be a major paper chase, and may be expensive, but it will clear the path for your future. The sooner you clean up your messes, the sooner you can succeed in life.

If you are debt free and have a savings account too, you're about as well-off as a person can expect to be. However, you may be frustrated to learn that through all your diligent saving and your abject denial of luxury, you may not qualify for assistance that is available to someone who has been more careless (No, the world is not a fair place). What you may be relieved to learn is that just because you have the money doesn't mean that you have to pay cash for your labor and delivery. You can work out a payment plan with most hospitals and midwives, and unlike credit cards, hospitals normally don't charge interest. Many people I know pay off their hospital bills at about $100.00 a month. Still, you must not miss a payment or it will end up on your credit report. In addition to this, most hospitals will be willing to bargain with you over the cost of your labor and delivery package, and they will take into consideration the fact that you are going to be a single mom, but sometimes you have to be pushy in order to get someone to talk to you about this. Talk to someone at the financial services office at your hospital. They might make you feel more at ease regardless of your financial picture.

Another Warning: **hospitals (as well as insurance companies) are notorious for screwing up your billing and charging a patient twice for services rendered**. Always check your hospital bills and make sure they are correct, even if you have to sacrifice in order to have enough time to do so! Midwives, on the other hand, usually offer more personalized service.

If the cost of your prenatal care, labor, and delivery are covered by your insurance, you are the luckiest dog of all. Still make a plan to get rid of your debts, pay all bills on time, and work at building savings accounts for both you and the baby.

Once you have taken a hard look at your financial situation you can begin to make a budget for your prenatal spending. Even future single mothers who are not worried about their finances can benefit through knowing what's available, what's necessary, and what they can expect in the way of prices. Keep in mind that there will most likely be a Baby Shower in your future, and that the most popular baby shower gifts are cute outfits and inexpensive necessities such as bottles and pacifiers. Read the next few sections, prioritize what you think is most important for your lifestyle, figure out what you can spend, stick to your limits, and have a great time shopping!

Financial Assistance

Even if you're not extremely worried about making ends meet, the fluff in your financial cushion will flatten a bit both while you are pregnant and thereafter. What you are going to do takes lots of money, and is usually paid for by more than one person. If you feel that you might need some help in this arena, there is absolutely no shame in getting extra assistance, so start looking for it as soon as possible. Some types of funding for your pregnancy and single motherhood are difficult to obtain, and some may have their drawbacks, but are sometimes necessary for your well-being.

Although assistance may come to you in many ways, there are a few things to remember about receiving this assistance. The first, which I call the "Golden Rule of Financial

Assistance," is this: Always be honest about your taxable income when filling out applications and receiving assistance. These programs are set up to help those in need, not those who merely want a free ride. Do not try to defraud the system. Not only will you be taking from those who need it, but you may face legal problems or be rendered incapable of receiving assistance in the future. In essence, you would be biting the hand that feeds you, and it's not very often that Uncle Sam does something out of the kindness of his heart. The second rule is this: Do not throw caution to the wind. Continue to be frugal with your money because the financial aid just might run dry, and there are always unexpected expenses and mistakes with purchases along the way.

Another thing that you must be prepared for when seeking assistance is this: Certain people who work in public assistance may assume that you're not very smart. Yes, this *is* incredibly insulting, but right now is not the time to waste your energy on it. The People at the Child Support Office (CSED) see so much drama, hysterics, and dishonesty that you may be perceived as just another body walking through the door trying to spitefully shake money out of the government because you haven't succeeded in shaking it out of the pockets of the man who dumped you. Your strategy is to play the game and do what you have to do to get what you need. You *need* that free paternity test. You *need* that free cereal and orange juice. If anyone implies or asks you something that is insulting, smile, shrug, laugh if you want to, and answer honestly. Do not give a joke answer, even if you think the answer is obvious, because that just might earn you a lecture and put you in a foul mood. Again, conserve your energy.

If ever you feel you have received extremely bad treatment from your case workers at WIC or CSED, write a letter after you no longer have to deal with them. I know it's hard, but swallow your pride and cooperate until then.

The WIC Program
The WIC Program (Women, Infants, and Children Program) is a nutritional program designed to help low-income women who may have difficulty sustaining their health through pregnancy because of lack of funding or knowledge. Even if you are well educated on nutrition and child care, it is a good idea to apply for WIC assistance to see if you qualify. And at this time, even organic foods are available through the WIC program, which wasn't the case when I was pregnant. If you know how to cook from scratch (see my book recommendation in **Chapter 7**), you will be eating as healthily as possible by using organic ingredients.

If you do qualify for WIC, the nutritionists and counselors will provide you with lots of information on your nutrition and health, will give you vouchers to help pay for some very important food items while you are pregnant, and will educate you on infant care issues. In addition, they will often come find you in the hospital and help you with learning to properly breastfeed your baby and answer any questions you might have. Something to keep in mind: although plans to breast feed are highly encouraged at WIC, failure or refusal to breast feed will not eliminate you from the program, and infant formula for your baby will be paid for by WIC after your baby is born. Always insist on formula that is organic or at least non-GMO.

If you do find yourself enrolled in the WIC Program, follow the rules of the program and keep your appointments. If you have more vouchers than you can use, stock up on non-perishables. Do not give your vouchers away. If you are overstocked, allow the occasional voucher to expire. The money in this program is intended to help needy mothers and children. If you can't use it yourself, leave it for another needy woman or child.

You can find the listing for your local WIC office through an Internet search.

Medicaid

If you don't have insurance and your income is low, you may qualify for Medicaid, which will greatly relieve the burden of your medical costs. When I was pregnant, in order to qualify for Medicaid, one must have had a low income and little or no money in a savings and checking account. I have since heard that the rules have changed, and that a woman's savings will no longer affect her ability to qualify for Medicaid (*Thank God*). However, as the rules have changed before, they may change again. Go to your local Medicaid office and fill out an application. If you are the right kind of applicant, you may end up paying nothing at all for the birth of your baby.

Other Insurance Programs

Some states have insurance and medical care programs for lower-income uninsured women who make too much money to qualify for Medicaid, or for children whose parents are uninsured. Again, each state has its own programs with their individual limits, and the availability of these programs changes often. Call your local Department of Health and Human Services in order to see if such a plan exists in your area.

Unemployment Insurance

Unemployment Insurance (most commonly referred to as "unemployment,") can be obtained if you are fired or laid off from a job you have had for a certain amount of time. You can apply for Unemployment Insurance and collect a certain amount of money for a limited time while you seek other employment. Do not hesitate to take advantage of this program. After all, you paid into it with your taxes. Contact your local Unemployment Insurance office listed in the government section of your phone directory.

Welfare and Food Stamps

The only way to know if you qualify for Welfare or Food Stamps is to go and apply. There is no shame in receiving Welfare if you need it, but remember that it should be regarded as only a temporary solution to a financial crisis. True, sometimes the odds are stacked against a woman and she cannot find a job for a long period of time regardless of how hard she tries, but anyone who actually plans to live off welfare for any length of time is doing a disservice to herself and to her country, and is hurting her baby's future as well. There are benefits and drawbacks to receiving welfare, as with any other assistance, and they vary from state to state (shockingly, some states require that welfare be paid back in the event that a welfare recipient ends up receiving child support from a baby-father who was previously un-contactable or who has recently found work). The benefits and drawbacks of Welfare in your home state can be explored with your caseworker.

Some Things New and Some Things Used

Yes, preparing for a baby is an expensive project, especially for those of us who plan to go it alone, but part of the fun of anticipating your baby is acquiring all that you will need. If you can afford to buy everything brand new, then you're one of the lucky few, but even those of you who are rolling in dough can use those extra ducats for a savings account, college fund, or for unexpected expenses down the road. You've got quite a while to prepare, and the expense of feathering your nest can be limited by your diligence.

Furthermore, buying used items is a habit that you can take into your future. While I am no longer hurting for money, I am still a careful shopper. If I try on a pair of expensive jeans at Nordstrom and happen to like them, I get the brand and style name and number, document them in my notes in my smartphone, and then look for them on e-bay. One of my favorite catalogues is very expensive. If I like an item, I know I will always eventually be able to find it on e-bay for a fraction of the price by searching the catalogue name, type of item (blouse, etc.), and size. Probably the best example of my saving was finding a $250 blouse for $12. Of course, sometimes you make a purchasing mistake. There are many ways you can address mistakes: re-list the item, take it to a consignment store, sell it at a garage sale, bring it to a clothing swap party, or—if you are making enough money that you need a tax write-off, donate it, save your receipt, and write it off your taxes.

Back to the baby: Certain personal items such as bottle nipples, thermometers, teething rings, and cloth diapers should always be purchased new, and some thought should go into the consistency of types and materials you wish for your baby to have, but make sure these products are free of Bisphenol-A or BPA. As awareness is increasing, BPA-free products are now easily identified and acquired through the internet if they're not available locally.

Anything else can be acquired for lower than normal prices at second-hand stores, on Craigslist.org, and sometimes the quality of the merchandise is much better than you had expected! Some new mothers are so overwhelmed and disorganized that certain clothes never even get used before they're on the rack at the thrift store, so the more you shop, the better your chances of hitting the "mother lode" (pun intended). Sometimes these same items can be found at Target or Fred Meyer at prices just as low as you would find in second hand stores, so be sure to check out what's available in the nearest super-store as well. And don't always spring for the cheapest item unless you know it's what you want.

If, before you have given these matters much thought, you are out shopping and find something you absolutely love and feel you can't live without, then by all means, get it! But first be aware of what quality items are available to you for free or at bargain prices before you go flattening your wallet on frivolities.

Bargains, Loaners, and Freebies

Read over the suggestions in these next few sections before you go shopping; and don't worry if you can't find everything you want right away for prices you can afford. Always hold out for the good stuff, and KNOW that the exact item that you want either is sitting in some shop somewhere in town, waiting for *you*, or its former owner just hasn't taken it to the thrift store or listed it on Craigslist yet. If you can't find what you want for the price you can afford, it will just have to go on your baby shower registry list.

Bargains

If you have a passion for finding a good deal, there are great deals everywhere, and you may find some veritable treasures hidden amidst the clutter and chaos of thrift stores, garage sales, or super-stores. Sites like Freecycle and Craigslist can supply you with sundry finds at a fraction of their original costs. Quality high-ticket items such as cribs, mattresses, strollers, car seats, swings, and changing tables can only be used for so long before the baby outgrows them, which means there is always a recycling supply in any city or small town. Second-hand buying, however, takes some time, diligence, and skill. Here are some tips that will help you weed through the thousands of items and discern what's a treasure and what's just trash.

Check for quality: Do your research on brand names, safety, and recalls. Ask salespeople what they know about a product, and ask them to demonstrate if they can. If an instruction manual is not included with the item, see if one can be obtained online or through the manufacturing company (sometimes the companies will charge you money to send you one, so don't assume that you can get one for free if you can't get one at the store). If the salesperson does not know about the items in question, ask when someone will be there who can help. Do not buy cribs made before 1992, as they might not adhere to modern safety standards.

Consider the costs of combined items: Some consignment stores will sell a crib and mattress together, which amounts in great savings to the buyer. Always check to make sure you're getting all that you expect from the price of an item.

Check for injuries: Make sure everything works the way it's supposed to. If it's broken, don't buy it, even if it seems like a bargain.

How's it going to clean up? Sometimes the greatest items go unnoticed because they are dirty. Check for detachable cloth parts that can be laundered or changed. Can the item in question be scrubbed down with scouring powder or painted with a safe, lead-free lacquer? If soil appears on plastic or metal parts of the object, it should clean up easily. *Always* wash everything you get for the baby, new or used.

Go thrift shopping in the ritzy part of town: The formula is simple: rich family buys best of everything brand new, baby outgrows them in same amount of time, rich neighborhood has fewer bargain hunters, and that's where *you* come in.

Check thrift stores frequently: Unlike department stores, thrift stores are not limited to when their shipments come in. You may strike gold on any lucky day.

Get to those garage sales early: Now that your late weekend nights are a thing of the past, make your mornings the time to hunt for bargains. Garage sales that feature baby items are usually listed on Craigslist or in the newspapers, so plan your route and get on the road!

Be sure to hit the library as well as second-hand book store: Second-hand book stores normally have a wide selection of books on everything you need to know, so make this a top priority early on in your pregnancy. Some popular books can be obtained through the Amazon.com "used copies" market, sometimes for the mere cost of shipping plus a dollar or two.

Whatever you do (and I say this as an author, knowing full well that I will not get a royalty each time one of my own books changes hands), from now on, do not buy new books if you can help it. Use the library as much as possible.

Loaners

Here is a list of some of the things you may be able to find on loan or rent for a reasonable price. Opportunities may vary from city to city.

Car Seats: ask your doctor about car seat check-out programs or rental programs through your doctor's office or hospital. He or she may refer to you your city police or department of transportation. We are warned never to buy a used car seat, but new car seats are always expensive. If the car seat you acquire is from a hospital or public safety program, it has been inspected and guaranteed to be safe. AND part of the deal just might be an installation demonstration from a cute cop or fireman (not a reason in itself, but certainly doesn't hurt).

Breast Pumps/ Breastfeeding Gear: Sometimes you can get these from your local WIC office. If not, contact your local chapter of La Leche League. They're always ready to assist expectant mothers who plan to bolster their babies' health and cut costs by breast feeding, and they can refer you to companies which rent or loan out top-of-the-line breast pumps. La Leche League in your area can be found through an internet search.

Books: most doctors' offices and midwives have a book check-out system with a great selection (this helps assure that the patients will pay their bills by making sure they don't spend all their money on books).

And again, do not forget about your local library. You can very often re-check a book several times, and if your library does not have a certain book in-house, they can often borrow the books that you need from another library. In addition, don't forget that you can also rent music and movies from the library. There's never any need to spend money on such things!

Freebies

You will acquire lots of free stuff throughout your pregnancy. Most of this stuff will come in the form of small but useful things such as free samples of shampoos, formulas, nursing pads, diapers, powders, etcetera. Be sure to keep like items together, and keep them organized and at easy reach so they will be convenient to use when you need them.

Again, make sure you go to the WIC office to see what you qualify for, and take everything that's offered. The friendly people at the WIC office will also occasionally give you free samples of useful magazines, nursing pads, and diapers, manual breast pumps, bottles… you name it! Your doctor's office might provide you with some fun surprises like diaper bags, videos, nursing pads, books, etc. If you opt for a hospital birth, make sure you leave with all the supplies in your room, because you will be charged for them regardless. You will normally acquire at least a nasal aspirator, thermometer, diapers, hemorrhoid cream, and baby wipes.

One of my favorite ways to get discounts and freebies is through loyalty programs at your local supermarket. These days the stores keep track of what you have bought and make offers based on what's going to bring you back to the store, and most of these loyalty programs have smartphone apps too, so you can check your offers while you are shopping rather than clipping coupons.

Making Extra Money for the New Addition

When making money is the issue at hand, a pregnant woman's motto is "seize the day," because one never knows what's around the corner. Even if you're financially "sitting pretty" at the time of your conception, you may find yourself panicked about your finances during the first six weeks of your baby's life or at some time in your pregnancy, especially if you are assigned to bed rest. It is obvious that anyone's financial situation can improve if she takes on a second job and fills her spare time with more work, but most pregnant women do not have the time or energy to do so during such a vulnerable time for their health and comfort, and you owe it to yourself to allow yourself to be pregnant.

One thing that is certain about the impending birth of your child is that your priorities are going to change drastically, and that money, time, and storage space will be right behind the baby in their levels of importance. Some extra funds can be acquired through the simple act of paring down, and doing so will benefit the expectant mother twofold because not only will she be acquiring extra cash, she will also be acquiring additional space, which always seems to shrink after the baby has arrived. In addition, you may get your share of exercise through the footwork that will accommodate any honest effort to effectively pare down.

Take an assessment of those items you will truly want and need, and try to liquidate the rest. Make sure you do so in your spare time, so as not to impinge on your job or other obligations and defeat the purpose of your efforts. Also be sure to avoid heavy lifting. If you are one of those people who has a strong attachment for "things," this is a good time to break this attachment: several studies have concluded that financial success if often closely connected to an individual's ability to sacrifice when necessary and to know what's important and valuable, and what's not!

Following are a few ideas on how to rid yourself of your excess baggage while earning a little treat for yourself.

Garage Sale

Having a garage sale is a lot of work, but if you have enough that needs to go, the work is worth it. You might want to advertise in the newspapers, but only if you feel that your profits will exceed the price of any advertising. Craigslist is best for putting up a free and easy ad, and that's where people look first these days. Always put up big easy-to-read weatherproof signs (I can't stress this enough. Make them Big, fluorescent, and cover them in Saran Wrap to protect them from the rain). It might be helpful to team up with a friend if you don't feel you have a wide enough range of things to sell, and please adhere to environmental garage sale etiquette and take your signs down when the sale is over. Those items that traditionally sell well are framed art, electronics, furniture, designer clothes in good condition, sporting goods, and baby items (not that you're going to be selling any of those, but it's good knowledge for the future). Whether or not you make good money can depend on everything from your signs to the weather, so put some energy into your preparation, be open to haggling, and cross your fingers and hope for a sunny day. If all else fails, it will be good practice for the *really* big garage sale you're going to have when your baby outgrows his newborn stuff.

Books
Most cities have used book stores that will give you cash or credit for your used books. Hang on to those books that you truly love and those college literature anthologies that get more expensive every year, and get rid of the rest (that pile of romance novels will just collect dust). If your local used book store won't take what you have, not all hope is lost…

Another way to get rid of your books is to establish a seller account at Amazon.com. This can, however, be time consuming, and if your books are extremely popular, you will have some stiff competition from those used booksellers who have a large inventory and can afford to part with their books for a dollar or two. Always consider Amazon's commission as well as how the shipping allowance compares to your actual shipping cost to see if it's really worth the effort for you.

If all else fails, the library may take them. If you donate books to the library, be sure to save the receipt and write the donation off your taxes.

Records, CDs, Videos, DVDs…
Most cities also have second-hand music and video stores that will buy your used Compact Discs. Again, don't sacrifice anything that is really special to you, as the money you receive for your discs will not be anywhere near what you paid for them, but if you bought that CD for one song you're now sick of or if you have it on iTunes, unload it.

Again, also consider getting a seller account at Amazon.com.

Clothes
It is also quite common these days to find vintage clothing stores and consignment stores that will be interested in selling some of your better used clothes. Jeans, well-kept formal gowns, antique garments, coats, jackets, and designer garments are normally good sellers. You'll have a better chance of getting what you want for them if you have a garage sale or attempt to sell items from certain trendy or classic designers, but if they're just taking up space, it's best to get rid of them. Keep in mind that consignment stores will normally give you a bigger cut of the profit than those buy-sell-trade places, but you will likely have to wait to get your money, and you might have to check back every week to see if any of your stuff has sold.

Again, eBay selling is an option for lightly used designer clothes. Always make sure to list where they came from (Sundance Catalog, Nordstrom, etc.,), brand name, item, size, and measurements.

I urge you, however, not to get rid of your most valuable and favorite clothes, even if you don't think you'll ever fit into them again. Pack them into a box, and take them out a year after your child is born. I got rid of all my pre-pregnancy clothes only to have to replace them year and a half after my son was born.

Collectibles

At the time this book was conceived, TY beanie babies were the hot commodity amongst collectors. I had acquired several of these at my baby shower, and inherited a few from friends who acquired them from McDonald's Happy Meals. I saved what I thought was the cutest one for my son and sold the rest—I made $225.00 in one hour.

Now, you might not want to do this with any family heirlooms or those special valuables that prove themselves over time, but if you are in possession of certain collectibles of which you are not a serious collector, you might want to see if they're worth more to someone else than they are to you. If you have access to a computer, learn to use eBay or another online auction site. You might also want to check the newspapers, or thumb through a collectors' magazine. You may be surprised at the value of what was shoved in the back of your closet.

Sporting Goods

Most sporting goods are rather expensive, but can thankfully be traded in at second-hand sporting goods stores for cash or credit. If those cross-country skis have been sitting in the back of your closet for four years and you live in Florida, do yourself (and someone else) a favor and trade them in. After all, if you haven't used them in years, it may be about four *more* years before your child offers you the mobility to plan a trip dedicated to using those skis.

Note: It is also a good habit to *buy* all of your sporting goods second-hand, particularly when you don't yet know if you are ready to commit to a sport. Remember this rule as your child grows and develops a "crush" on a different sport each season.

Handmade and Vintage

Word on the street is that artisans can sell their crafts on a site called Etsy.com. I have also come to understand that unlike eBay, selling on Etsy.com does not require that you adhere to a certain time line, as one would when using an auction site. In addition, their fees are far more reasonable. If you have several pieces of vintage apparel, or if you are an artisan or a seamstress, Etsy.com may be the perfect way to market and sell your wares.

I have to add an extra endorsement for sites such as Etsy.com and on-line auction sites, as they do so many things to help our local economy: First of all, they eliminate the middle man, putting the power directly into the hands of those who make or find the desired goods: People just like you and me. They diminish our relationship with and support of companies that rely on third-world countries that exploit their workforce in order to boast low prices. Using sites like these is better for the environment: There is less shipping, packaging, and transportation than when we purchase from ANY store. Purchasing crafts and clothes from Etsy.com is a lot like going to your local farmer's market: It is an act of good karma. Do, however, always check for product and seller reviews and do lots of comparison shopping: Quality can vary widely.

Put an ad in the paper
Many newspapers have "freebies" sections which might give you free advertising for your "for sale" items which cost $100.00 or less. If your local newspaper has such an offer, take advantage of it.

Have a "paring down" party
There will always be great items which were rejected by the owner of the local consignment store or just didn't get bought from your garage sale, but because you had decided to part with them, you had fallen out of love with these things, secure in the thought that they would make you some money, which is important to you right now. You might also be tired of lugging things all over town while trying to get them sold. Rest easy—*there is still a chance!* Invite your friends over and have a "Paring Down" party or a clothing swap party (also known as a "naked lady party" when the traded items are mostly clothes. At these parties, it is customary to wear underwear you're not afraid to be seen in, because everyone's in a trying-on frenzy)! Let everyone know that they can also bring things that they can trade, and give everyone great deals on the things you no longer want. True, you may make nothing at all, but you'll have a good time doing it!

Be an online auction entrepreneur
You know that pair of Dansko clogs you bought for a dollar at your neighbor's garage sale will get you sixty if you sell them on online. Those English pub towels your ex-boyfriend left behind will get you fifteen. Those Vampire costumes you've kept since college are in high demand with the Goth crowd these days, and that itchy Norwegian sweater you can't stand to wear is worth two hundred dollars to someone else. If you have stuff lying around that no longer has any use to you, it can be turned into on-line auction gold. Yes, it does take time to list them, a camera of some kind is necessary, you do have to answer lots of buyer questions, and you do have to box things up and take them to the

post office, but when you see that you've earned an extra hundred or two dollars at the end of the month, it might be worth it!

A word of warning: If an item cannot be sold for more than ten dollars, your listing might not be worth your investment (to list your item will cost somewhere between three and ten dollars). Do some preliminary research to see what like items are selling for, and pay attention to how long they've been listed and whether or not they have any bids.

Put it on Craigslist
Most everyone these days knows about Craigslist.org, but if you don't, *run* to your computer this instant and check it out! Not only can you *get* things on Craigslist, you can also *get rid of* practically anything! Unlike eBay, it costs nothing to put an ad on Craigslist. Pay attention to the rules though. Certain things (such as pets) cannot be sold on Craigslist, and many listings are simply ignored. For example, craigslist is a great place to sell furniture or a bicycle, but the listings for certain collectibles will collect cyber-dust on Craigslist and will be better off listed on eBay, so make sure there is actually a market for what you are listing where you are listing it.

What do I do with all this left-over stuff?
Okay, we have to face the fact that some things are just junk, but some things are not! If you feel that something has value, box it up, and put it out of the way. Of all the stuff that you have decided is not worth keeping around, donate the stuff that is still usable to Salvation Army, Red Cross, or any other charity (keep in mind that even thrift stores don't want things that are not in good condition—no holes, no stains, no broken parts—otherwise, they end up in the landfill. Throw broken things away or give them to someone interested in restoring them, and cut up old clothes and use them as cleaning rags). Make sure you ask for a receipt, and write the value of the items off your taxes as a charitable contribution. Some charities have pick-up service. If you need things to be picked up, make sure the driver will give you a receipt or that you can otherwise get one.

Resist the Urge vs. Time to Splurge
Although you can cut costs at certain corners, you cannot (nor should you) get *everything* second-hand, and you would be wise to allow yourself some financial leeway with certain goods and services.

This next section explores the ways that you can be strategic with your purchases throughout your pregnancy.

Resist the Urge (in other words, try not to buy):

1. Anything you're not sure will fit
Do not go shopping for non-maternity clothes after your fourth month. In doing so, you are liable to spend money on something that may or may not fit after your baby's born. Adversely, don't buy any maternity clothes (aside from underwear, bras, and hosiery as needed) until after you start to grow. You might be surprised to find that your chest and thighs change size as well, and the items you bought at the beginning of your pregnancy might be too small.

2. Too many baby clothes
Trust me: Your baby will have enough clothes. He or she might even have too many. You will probably find that many of the cuter items you have acquired will be worn only once or twice, as you will learn that many things are hard to get on and off or that they are uncomfortable. Most everyone you know will get you something for the baby to wear. If you find one or two outfits that really inspire you, go ahead and get them, but don't break the bank on the baby's wardrobe.

3. A New Dog or Cat
New pets are generally a no-no for single pregnant women because they add extra responsibility and expense to a situation that is already going to create a strain on your free time and your finances. In addition, it is impossible to know what your child is or isn't going to be allergic to, and it's always heartbreaking to have to get rid of an animal you have bonded with, even if it's for the sake of your child. I myself had to give up my beloved cat after we found my son was allergic—thankfully, my parents were able to take her, so it wasn't like we had to part ways, but it was a huge sacrifice not to have her in my everyday life. If you live in a rural area with lots of space that doesn't get too warm or too cold for year-round outdoor pets (and you're sure you can find another comparable home if you need to), you might have more freedom than most of my audience to make a commitment to a new animal. However, if you live in an urban area, don't press your luck. Wait until you know what life as a parent is going to look like before you get a new dog or cat.

If you want something to come home to, consider getting a bird or a goldfish—They require less time, money, and energy than a dog or cat does. Exotic pets often require a consistent temperature and a special diet, so I would warn against an animal whose food you couldn't buy at the supermarket, or who might freeze to death if your power goes out. If you crave the companionship of a dog during your daily walks, you can offer to walk a neighbor's dog, or advertise as a dog walker and work your walking time around your schedule. You may end up with all of the assets of pet ownership without any of the drawbacks.

Time to Splurge:

1. These days, you need a smartphone. I'm sure I don't need to sell you in the idea that you need a smartphone: Camera, email, text, music, bills and banking, social media, transportation apps, shopping apps, maps, clock, weather, notes, meditation apps, etc., are all at your fingertips. Of course, having all this magic at your command can also be a curse! Please read **Chapter 7** and take steps to ensure that your smartphone is truly your ally rather than an informant through your pregnancy and motherhood journey and beyond.

2. *The second-most important baby gear item is a computer.*
While your first priority may be to have a smartphone, the computer has other, more homey roles than either a smartphone or a tablet. Most importantly (in my opinion), storing photos, word processing/ writing and storing resumes and other important documents (never delete outdated resumes—you may have to look at past jobs to prove your qualifications in a field you never thought you'd be working in), copying and reproducing music and audio files from discs, enhancing career prospects or performing work at home, playing games, applying for jobs, printing photographs or other materials (which, of course, depends on you: there are many places that provide printing services, so if you don't do it often, a printer is not necessary), etc., are all invaluable conveniences for a busy single parent who has no choice but to spend a lot of time in the house. A computer can help you multi-task, which you will be doing a lot of over the next two or three years. You can set your computer to the task of finding information, get up, change the baby, come back to the computer, put the dinner on, look at the computer, fold laundry… this beats budgeting a whole day to find a map, buy a book, go shopping for cloth diapers, buy a newspaper, and trying to make it home in time to see your favorite TV show. In the good old days, one could never expect to do all of these things in one day. In my opinion, a computer (with Microsoft Office loaded in it) is more important than most of what our society would have you believe is important. If you don't have one, why not put one on your baby shower registry and let everyone know that this is what you need? Furthermore, it is easier on your eyes and your neck *not* to be on the smartphone all day long.

3. *Comfortable shoes are not a luxury—they're a necessity!*
When it comes to shoes, don't even *think* about sacrificing comfort for savings. Your feet are two of the most important things you own. Sure, some people have extremely

adaptable feet, but if you're not one of these people (and I am *not)*, be kind to yourself and make sure your shoes are comfortable. There is a perfectly good reason that certain shoes are so expensive—it's because they look good and are comfortable at the same time. If you want stylish and comfortable shoes and are on a budget, check out Aerosoles. Many of their prices are competitive with those of discount shoe stores, and you are guaranteed a comfortable product. Some of the shoes (and styles) don't have a lot of "staying power," but they will be comfortable for as long as they last. Dansko brand shoes are more classic and last longer, but are also more costly.

3. *Spare no expense on the best stroller for your needs!*
If you can find exactly what you want and need at a discount, that's just great. If you can't, you might as well bite the bullet and get exactly what you want, regardless of the cost. Good strollers have great re-sale value, and a stroller is one of those things that helps assure your freedom and autonomy, and improves the quality of your life.

4. *Go ahead and treat yourself to a pedicure.*
While you are pregnant, your feet will be hard to reach, and they will be carrying more weight than they're used to. They're likely to be sore, calloused, stressed, and have probably looked much better at other times in your life. Hunt around for the best combination of price and service, and go ahead and treat yourself to a pedicure. After all, making your feet feel better is something probably you can't do on your own right now.

5. *A haircut from a trusted professional will help lighten your load!*
While you are pregnant, you will have no control over certain aspects of your appearance. One exception is your hair. Sure, there are more important things in life than your appearance, and nobody knows that better than you right now, but taking pride in your appearance does not mean that you are superficial, self-critical, desperate, or anti-feminist. Your body is a temporary shelter for your soul, and it is up to you to arrange the furniture the way it pleases you.

Personal tastes vary, but you have only yourself to impress. If you feel like you look your best with long, flowing, unkempt hair, then keep it that way, but if you feel best with a more modern and precise cut, please don't break out the shears and take hair matters into your own hands—you will regret it!

For most women, now is not the time to do anything drastic: don't go super short if you have long hair, don't cut bangs if you've never had them before, and don't experiment with a wild color unless it's something you do regularly and your job doesn't depend on your having a conservative appearance.

6. Professional movers are worth their weight in gold.
If you find yourself needing to relocate while you're pregnant (or while you have a baby or toddler) and you don't have a gang of strong friends and relatives who want to help you for free, don't hesitate to hire professional movers. No matter where you live, there will be one or two small moving companies that boast reasonable prices for getting your life moved from point A to point B. Professional movers will move you more quickly and efficiently than your friends will, and you won't have to worry about anything or anyone (including yourself) getting hurt—all you have to do is box all your stuff up. Remember to tip your movers if you feel you were given great service (don't worry about how much—every little bit is appreciated), and remember who they are in case you ever need them again.

7. Stretch marks last a long time—do they have to be there at all?
If the women in your family have a history of developing stretch marks, it is wise to invest in a preventative treatment for them. Such treatments in the form of lotions and oils in a variety of price ranges can be found at maternity stores or department stores. There is no solid proof that these products work no matter how much they cost, but hey, if you don't want stretch marks, they're definitely worth a try.

This is a true stretch mark story from yours truly, and these stretch mark preventative measures won't cost you any more money than using lotion: As one who doesn't have a genetic predisposition for developing stretch marks, I wasn't extremely worried about it, but I used **St. Ives Collagen and Elastin Lotion** (available at most supermarkets) on my belly, aware that elastin makes skin more resilient. Well, the day after my son was born and I could see my whole body for the first time in months, I noticed that I had indeed developed stretch marks, but only in the area under my pubic hair. Were my stretch marks a result of said area not having received lotion, or had said area stretched during labor, out of eyeshot of their hostess? I will never know for certain, but you can take from this story whatever you wish, for every word of it is true.

Anyway, if you develop stretch marks despite your commitment to using stretch mark products, just accept the fact that you have a genetic predisposition to get them, remind yourself that it could be worse, and remember that any suitor who would decide against liking you because of stretch marks is truly just a scumbag who is not worth your time.

8. Good food (It makes life worth living!)
Life in America certainly has its benefits, but it has its drawbacks as well. As discussed in **Chapter 2**, one of the less obvious drawbacks is that our nation's food supply is... well... filthy. The ground beef you buy at the grocery store is usually the product of thousands of cows, some of them too sick to walk, going through a grinder that by law only has to

be cleaned at the end of the day. The milk you buy at the grocery store is often full of antibiotics, which have led to dangerous resistant bacteria; and Bovine Growth Hormone (rBGH or rBST), the effects of which have not been fully studied, but is linked to the fact that so many American children are overweight despite their being sufficiently active. Most national and grocery store brands include genetically modified ingredients that are banned in Europe and Japan, and were never tested by the FDA because of a decision made by our "brilliant" former vice president, Dan Quayle. Sadder still, one of the most popular brands of baby formula in the U.S. uses the genetically-engineered ingredients that are banned in other countries. These days, most everyone knows that the pesticides on our fruits and vegetables can cause all sorts of horrible things to happen to our bodies, not to mention our earth and our water supply.

Another disheartening fact: At one time in history, one could often safely assume that a person was skinny because he or she was too poor to overeat. Interestingly, these days the same can be said for someone who is overweight: The cheaper the food, the more likely it has empty calories, pesticides, edible food-like substances, Trans fats, GMOs, and very little nutritional value. Most people live closer to a convenience store than to an actual supermarket, yet one can't find the components of a true healthy meal at a convenience store.

Yes, natural and organic foods are expensive, but sometimes if you keep your eyes open, you can find good deals on certain items at farmers' markets or at your local grocery store. And if you get into the habit of buying and eating produce on a regular basis, not only will you be healthier, but your bank account will be healthier too. As discussed before, If you are a meat eater, try to find meats raised without hormones or antibiotics (this is especially important for ground beef). If you drink milk, look for an organic alternative, or at least one that doesn't have growth hormones. If you feed your baby formula, you can't go wrong by investing in organic formula. Healthy grocery buying can indeed be expensive, but you might be saving yourself money slated for future medical costs. You might not be able to do it all the time, but it's wise to try to do it when you can. After all, what you put in your body builds up in your body. Good food is medicine, and bad food is poison. You and your baby deserve to be healthy and to live a long, productive, rewarding, successful life. If it's within your means, it is worth the expense.

9. *Underwear, hosiery, and bras*
The moment your body starts to itch and stretch, you'll want to give it room. You will probably be surprised at how quickly and drastically your bra size will change, and you might want to get fitted at a department store—When the sales clerk told me that I should start wearing a 36 D-cup (when I started I was a 32 B), I was in shock and wondered if

she knew what she was talking about, but as soon as I changed my bra, I was breathing a nice, roomy sigh of relief. I'm still not sure it fit properly, but I didn't care—I was comfortable.

Ditto for the underpants and hosiery. Yes, pregnancy pants may be ugly, but they'll be your best friends as soon as you meet. Always graduate to the next size if they leave marks on your body when you take them off.

Again, don't sacrifice comfort for a bargain. Bras and underwear can be expensive, but you are not helping yourself at all when you buy the two itchy cheap bras when you could have bought one more expensive, but much more comfortable bra. Go for comfort at all costs.

What you do and don't need will depend largely on your lifestyle, your support network, your living space, and your personal preference, but I hope these suggestions have helped you to think it over and come up with a list of your own potential urges to resist and splurges not to kick yourself over. Although it's always good to be thrifty, I feel that you should never deny what's necessary for the sake of saving a dollar or two. Remember, you're number one. If you sacrifice to the point that life is unbearable, that's what your life will be—unbearable! It is your right as an individual to make an assessment of what is going to help you live the happy, stress-free life you deserve.

Chapter Six

The Symbiotic Relationship between Child Support and Custody

The question of whether or not to seek child support is one of the most controversial, confusing, and potentially frustrating topics for single mothers-to-be. Sometimes single pregnant women question whether or not they're entitled to child support, especially in the event that the fathers of their children question or deny paternity. Thankfully, every custodial parent is considered entitled to child support—a paternity denial does not change that. However, depending on the circumstances surrounding the relationship between the mother and father of the child, the mother may decide that seeking child support is not worth the risks of including the child's father in her life if she will be compromising with visitation and custody.

Sadly, there are no straight answers to many questions about child support—they depend on a combination of the individuals involved and how they conduct themselves, the state in which the child is (or will be) born, and the personal values of any judges involved in legal proceedings (which I hope you are able to avoid if possible, as court can be costly and frustrating). Although in some states, a man who has had little or no contact with a woman throughout her pregnancy is not likely to be able to get any rights whatsoever; in some states, a combative or even dangerous and destructive man who has been absent for years can petition for paternity, visitation, or custody, walk into a woman's life, and take a child he has no idea how to care for away from its mother for a weekend, or even successfully arrange to get partial custody.

Given this diversity, it is extremely important that a mother-to-be do her research on the state in which she lives and thoroughly evaluate her circumstances in order to make the best decision she can. Having helped hundreds of women through this process, I have found that the best way to assist you is in evaluating your situation is making sure you understand your situation fully. This first part (this chapter) requires understanding child support and custody laws, trends, and social climates, and evaluating the benefits and risks of your situation. The second part (**Chapter 7**) involves knowing how to communicate with your child's father in order to keep yourself legally and personally safe. Please read both chapters before you initiate contact with your baby's father.

First, I am going to give you an important assignment for you to complete in the next few days: Do an internet search for your home state. Search, for example, "Child support guidelines Alaska," "Father's rights Alaska," "Unwed mother's rights Alaska," and "Child Custody Alaska." Call your local Child Support Services Division, and find out what they can tell you about the child support and custody laws in your area: Find out who must pay for the paternity test, find out how much of the father's income will be owed if paternity is confirmed, and find out whether the father has any automatic rights (other than the right to seek visitation or custody through court) if paternity is confirmed. Additionally, find out how much time a child's father would have to be absent in order for the child to be deemed "abandoned" and his rights terminated (and don't be surprised if they simply don't know—lots of people, despite working in the field, do not have a complete education on the current social climate). Also find out if your state has a Family Law Help Center or similar where you can file paternity paperwork, request emergency child custody orders, or file a parenting plan in the event that your child's father is being cooperative.

Again, please also read **Chapter 7** before you continue or establish communication with your child's father, as these two chapters may permanently change the way you communicate through your new awareness of the potential consequences of flippancy or emotionally-charged correspondence.

Legal Terminology in Plain Speak:
Child abandonment
Legally, in most states, a parent is said to have "abandoned" a child—and their parental rights are terminated—after a two-year period of withholding his or her contact and financial support when the custodial parent has not blocked access.

Child support
The money a non-custodial parent pays to the custodial parent in order to maintain the child's needs

Joint custody
When both parents of a child have equal rights and responsibilities (both are custodial parents)

Joint legal custody
When both parents of a child are expected to work together to make decisions for a child, including where the child goes to school, medical decisions, etc.

Joint physical custody
When a child has equal time and access to both parents' houses

Legal custody
The decisions regarding where a child goes to school, what medical care the child receives, what traditions are embraced

Physical custody
The right to decide where the child physically lives

Parenting/ co-parenting plan
A plan filed with the courts that outlines the roles and responsibilities each parent agrees to (this is a new legal trend, and should be implemented in any co-parenting arrangement)

Paternity
The proof—either through the signing of the birth certificate, a signed declaration in the form of a paternity affidavit, or genetics test—that a man is a child's father

Primary caregiver
The person who is providing for the majority—if not all—of a child's needs

Shared custody
When both parents have rights, but one parent has slightly more authority than the other, usually based on the schedule of where the child most often stays overnight. (Although this sounds like it could be a good deal, it is often difficult to enforce the decisions of the custodial parent)

Sole custody
The exclusive right and responsibility to care for a child

Sole legal custody
The exclusive right and responsibility to make decisions for a child

Sole physical custody
The exclusive right and responsibility to provide a home for a child

Supervised visitation
The right to see a child in the presence of a legal chaperon

Visitation
The right to visit a child whether in or away from the child's home

Where do I start?
Your friends and family may all have heard conflicting information about your rights as a parent and what's likely to happen. Sadly, just as every state and every situation differs, it is impossible to keep up with all the changes in laws and how they will affect you. For that reason, you will have to do some of this research on your own, find the sweet spot between what you want and what seems realistic, and make a solid plan.

Another frightening fact is that while women who were married to a man often make out like bandits—and if you do any dating of divorced men you will hear all about how unfair the legal system has been to them regarding their rights as fathers—women who become pregnant out of wedlock aren't often given this consideration. Yup, here come those patriarchy rules again—you failed to follow them. This puts extra weight on your behavior in any communication and legal proceedings, as you may very easily be perceived as the troublemaker.

But back to the point: You need to start with evaluating 1) what it is that you want, 2) whether or not it is likely/realistic, 3) whether it is recommended, 4) if it is what your child's father seems to want as well, and 5) how you can get it.

Here are some options for how you might answer the question, "What do I want?"

> I want my child's father to get back together with me and for us to be a family
>
> I want to have a peaceful co-parenting relationship with my child's father with equal participation, cooperation, and compromise from both parties.
>
> I want my child's father to be involved in my child's life and to pay child support, but I do not want him to have the right to affect my life or parenting decisions.

I will leave the door open for my son's father to come back into our child's life as a parent, but only for a certain amount of time because I want to be able to move forward in life without baggage or ties.

I want my child's father essentially out of our business, but I still want child support.

I am so certain my child's father will be a physical danger or economic liability to us that I want him gone, and the child support is not worth it.

Now let's define those wants in legal terms:

"I want my child's father to get back together with me and for us to be a family." (Marriage)

"I want to have a peaceful co-parenting relationship with my child's father with equal participation, cooperation, and compromise from both parties." (Joint custody)

"I want my child's father to be involved in my child's life and to pay child support, but I do not want him to have a significant effect on my life or parenting decisions." (Shared custody with mother as the custodial parent, and full paternal visitation rights)

"I will leave the door open for my son's father to come back into our child's life as a parent, but only for a certain amount of time—if I get a new husband, I want him to be able to adopt my child." (Sole custody, eventually terminating paternity rights due to child abandonment)

"I want my child's father essentially out of our business, but I still want child support." (Sole custody with paternity established, possible visitation)

"I am so certain my child's father will be a physical danger or economic liability that I want him gone, and the child support is not worth it." (sole custody, child abandonment)

"I want my child's father's agreement that he wants nothing to do with this, and set us both free forever—I do not plan to ever seek child support." (signing away paternal rights)

Now you should ask yourself, "Does what I want seem to respect the free will of everyone involved?" For example, if you want marriage, but your son's father is not interested or is already married to someone else, you will likely have to accept that marriage is not something both parties seem to want, or at least be ready for. If you want your son's father to sign away his paternal rights but he has been clear he wants to be a father to his child and has made attempts to communicate effectively with you, asking him to sign away his rights is potentially very hurtful to the possibility of being civil in the future and just might start an unnecessary war. If you want your son's father to be involved in your child's life, but—like the above example—he is not doing his part, you have to choose from a more realistic option, and one that does not compromise your rights as the one committed parent.

Interpreting whether a plan of action will honor a person's free will involves taking an assessment of both their words and actions.

Are his words and actions aligned?

Following are some scenarios that can be clear or confusing, and what you may choose to do about it.

Aligned negative:

He says he doesn't want to be involved and hasn't contacted you.

1. He knows about the pregnancy but hasn't said anything and hasn't contacted you.
2. He has asked you to stay away from him.
3. He has denied the possibility of paternity publicly or privately.
4. He has avoided or cut off communication and has blocked you on social media/ left you no way of getting in touch with him.
5. He has spoken about you to others in a destructive or damaging way.

These are examples of men whose words and actions both clearly demonstrate that they do not want the responsibility of the child. It is not recommended to insist upon more responsible behavior from men such as these. These scenarios empower the mother to press ahead with plans of sole custody as well as abandonment if she so desires. In the event that the mother plans to seek child support, there is a greater chance that she will not compromise her status as sole custodian, but it helps to save documentation of evidence of any of the above situations, as men often flip-flop about what they want when paternity is confirmed or a woman seeks child support. Sometimes men like these make false claims about the woman's actions in order to support their mission ("She pushed me away." "I tried to get in touch with her."), but they will likely fail if the woman saves evidence of documentation (again, please read **Chapter 7** before you continue or initiate any contact with the baby's father).

Aligned positive:

1. He says he does want to be involved and has reached out to communicate with you in a non-threatening way.
2. He insists on being in the child's life and is being very pushy about it, won't stop calling or writing, is bugging your friends, etc., but has not been violent or made threats.

This is an example of a person whose words actions are aligned to show that he wants to be a father to the baby. This is a situation in which joint or shared custody may be viable.

When a person's words and actions are not aligned, it is much more difficult to figure out whether or not your plans are aligned with their free will. However, in my opinion, people who subscribe to this type of behavior are very often what I refer to as energy stealers: They like the attention and energy that they get from stirring up drama, and they either don't know or don't care how damaging it can be to other people involved. In other words, they are not worried about your free will, so they are forfeiting your consideration in the process. Following are examples with my commentary.

Not Aligned:

1. He says he wants to be involved in the child's life but has been insulting, verbally abusive, coercive, gossipy, or flaky.
    My opinion: Dangerous. Potential verbal or physical abuser. Do not fool yourself into believing a co-parenting relationship can work well with this person, at least not at this time. Protect yourself.
2. He has encouraged you to have an abortion, but is saying that if you have the baby, he will "take the baby away from you."
    My opinion: See answer from number 1.
3. He says he doesn't want the baby/want a serious relationship with you, but continues to be sentimental, romantic, or affectionate and/or maintains contact with you.
    My opinion: Whatever you do, don't ever believe he is boyfriend material. This one likes to take your energy. He is not capable of understanding how much energy a baby takes.

Are *your* words and actions aligned?

As you continue this process, always make sure that your own words and actions are aligned as well. This includes:

If the father truly wants to be involved in the child's life, do not play games or withhold contact out of vengeance or to make the father squirm. Preventing a person from resolution of problems or keeping them away from their family can be maddening, and can turn them into a monster. If a person is willing to play fair (see next chapter to understand what that means), is not dangerous or abusive, and truly wants to be involved, it is best to give him a road map of how that can be accomplished in a way that is fair to you. If you are not ready to hash out the details of what is needed in order to have productive relations (again, see next chapter), let him know that he is not shut out, but that you need time to work out the terms that will be fair.

Do not withhold contact simply because you have decided you are not romantically interested in the father or you have lost your attraction or connection. You don't have to be interested in someone in order for him to be a good father. Single mothers-to-be get understandably itchy when the topic of father's rights comes up, so please understand what is being said here: If the father is *willing to play fair*, it is not fair to the child to alienate him from a loving parent. A man does not have to be what you want in order to be what the child wants.

Please don't play games. Don't do hurtful things in order to stir up drama when you know the baby's father is not interested in leaving. You don't want drama to become the habit. Stabbing holes in each other will only turn two potentially strong parents into pieces of energetic Swiss cheese. Always keep your intentions productive for your child. When a parent is committed to a child, that parent belongs to that child. Don't destroy your child's assets.

Remember that it is never a good idea to try to make a person walk a path he is not willing to walk. You can sometimes get someone to do what you want for a period of time, but if to do so is not their true choice, it often ends tragically and explosively. Furthermore, it is never the highest level of ethics to block someone's access to something they are committed to taking good care of.

If your child's father has been coercive, insulting, verbally (or physically) violent, indecisive, too casual, or chronically avoidant, then all bets are off: I am hoping that in these cases you will be wise enough not to hand him any rights or responsibilities he hasn't demonstrated the desire or ability to handle.

Now that we have examined everyone's motives and behavior, let's revisit our legal terminology and analyze what your wants and options are:

Marriage: This would have to be agreed upon by both parents.

Joint (physical and legal) Custody: You must both be people who are interested in parenting and must be extremely cooperative with each other, as it takes an extreme situation to reverse joint custody. If one parent makes much more money than the other, there may be some child support ordered.

Shared custody (with mother as custodial parent): The father will ideally have to demonstrate interest in being a parent and his willingness to pay child support, and it is ideal that the two parents agree upon most parenting issues. In this situation it is always best to file a parenting or co-parenting plan, as cooperation and agreement between parents can come and go with the seasons.

Sole custody with child support and unsupervised visitation: This is often established when the father has not demonstrated a consistent interest in being a parent, while also not demonstrating that he is a physical danger to the mother or child (although he may be an economic liability), but has made an admission or confirmation of paternity. In some cases, parties peacefully agree that this is the best arrangement for their careers and the child's stability. Often a good way to ensure you get sole custody is to 1) make sure the father has your contact information, 2) refrain from engaging in any drama or argumentative behavior, and 3) refrain from making any demands of him.

Sole custody as the result of the father not being involved in any way in your life or the child's life: While people often have judgments about this situation, I have no such judgments. Some women never disclose the identities of their babies' fathers and say they are unknown, some simply don't know who they are, sometimes the mother doesn't know the father's last name and can't find him, and sometimes the fathers of the babies are even dead. When the child's father is unknown, all custody reverts to the mother.

Sole custody as the result of child abandonment: If a child's father is not contactable for a certain amount of time (depends on the state), some states will deem the child abandoned, and all custody will be awarded to you—however, in cases such as this, you will not get child support. In order for this to work, some states require that you demonstrate that you have left the door open for contact with the child's father. Some judges even go so far as require you to give him a warning of your plans, if possible. Because of this, it is important to document dates and modes of communication, and to have them in writing. However, in some cases, the fact that you have been the only one caring for this child is enough.

Things to keep in mind while you come up with your plan
Remember: you can never choose a path for someone else. You can show them the path, but you can't make them walk it. If you want your child's father to be a part of your lives but he is not interested enough to follow protocol, you have to detach from his path and walk your path without him, and you can't depend on whether he ever catches up with you. In the next chapter I will show you a way to communicate with him to find out if he is interested in cooperating with you at all. If he is not willing to be fair or demonstrate responsibility, it is important that you position yourself so that he cannot wreck the stability that you have established.

Although we all know that emotional abuse is an extreme situation, the way our society works, women are still often blamed for an associated man's emotional misbehavior. Do not expect the courts to see things like they are. Play it smart in order to get what you want.

If your child is the result of your being the victim of one of the more recognized forms of extreme abuse (rape, incest, violence), you still have the right to keep your baby if that is your choice. Many counselors or other people in your life will assume that you don't want to, and that you are only considering abortion or adoption. If you have decided that you want to keep and be a mother to your baby, it is nobody's business where that baby came from. Of course, that won't prevent people from asking about it. Using phrases like, "the father is not involved," or "it's in the past and I have moved on," are good ways to close the door to that conversation without investing too much of your energy into it and without having to make up a lie you need to keep up with. Unevolved people love to judge other people's situations, so if your situation is something you have to explain in order for you or your child to be welcomed and treated fairly, learn ways to minimize the exchange of information. Although some people say that children born of these situations "carry sins" or some other nonsense, keep in mind that every person on earth is very likely the result of someone having been raped at one time or another. Incest—as horrible as it is—is something that has happened throughout the history of the world. The circumstances that lead to a child's existence are not that child's fault or doing. He or she does not "carry the sins" of any other person.

Don't say it if you don't mean it. I often see women's "final" letters to the fathers of their babies, and many times they say something like, "You don't have to be a part of this if you don't want to—I will take care of everything, but I want you to be a part of the baby's life if you want, so the door is open to you." I myself did this when I found out I was pregnant. Although this may seem mature and forgiving, look harder: Not only is it manipulative (it's offering yourself to be used as a doormat with the hope and belief that he will not take you up on it), but as time goes by, it is very unlikely that you will be okay with this situation! Saying you will take on the entire burden of a child in order to make a father feel comfortable meandering in every once in a while is economically unfair to you, and also may not be fair to your child.

Remember: To block information is always better than to lie, if it is possible. As someone who is on your side, I understand the desire to paint a rosier picture of your situation if it is something that people will judge, or if it's something that hurts for you to think about. However, if you make up stories, you will have to remember them. I've heard everything from "he's dead" to "he raped me," and then the story changes later, and there can be social or legal consequences.

However, there are also situations where a woman must "go there" to keep herself safe. "I don't know who the father is" is something that can earn you a ration of judgment, but it can also protect you from having to jump through legal hoops that may compromise your safety. If you find this to be your best option, brace yourself for the fallout, and only say this if it becomes necessary (don't tell one friend the truth and another friend the story—you will never be able to have them both in the same room again). If a person's intention is to have a functional friendship with you, they will often settle with "he's out of the picture," or "he wasn't ready to be a father." Bonus: If you plan to have a relationship in the future, good men respect a woman who can demonstrate this boundary without exposing all the details—it shows that she is empowered to make good decisions for herself. You have years before you will need to explain things to your child, so don't worry about that right now.

Is it okay to lie to the government? In my opinion, that depends on the situation. I personally feel that the government often asks questions that are nobody's business and that compromise a person's safety. You may be familiar with the "Trail of Tears," when the Federal government deported the Cherokee, Chickasaw, and Choctaw people from their ancestral homeland in Tennessee and surrounding states, forcing them to walk to Oklahoma (many of them barefoot), where they were not even familiar with how to farm the land—many died on the trip. The first part of this process was for all the people in the tribe to sign their names on the rolls to document that they were in fact Native American. Being members of their tribes and being unaware of the government's plan, most of them had no problem formally admitting this, and encouraged their families and tribe members to do the same. What they didn't know is that they were giving the government information on exactly who to deport.

This is a similar situation to when people imply that you're being dishonest when you don't chase a man down the street telling him exactly what he needs to do to be listed on your child's birth certificate. It will be easier to get child support if the child's father is listed on the birth certificate, but it will be harder to travel internationally without that father's approval. It will in a sense bind you to request his cooperation for you to live your life with your own child in tow, and will formally demonstrate his cooperation, willingness, or desire to be a father, even if he does nothing else.

Note: There will be many birth certificate discussions throughout this book—be careful about how you address this important issue.

The social climate of where you live: Single Mother-Friendly, or Single Mother-Hostile?

Laws vary from state to state, and court outcomes vary from judge to judge. Although it is important to learn whether your state laws and social climate are friendly or hostile to mothers, it is equally important that you not take any outcome for granted, and that you continue to put all your protections in place.

What is a single mother-friendly social climate? A single pregnant woman can often tell when she is going to have more than her share of push-back for a decision to keep her baby. Her social climate is made up by her friends, family, co-workers, state laws, and elected leaders.

A single mother-friendly legal climate is one in which a child's father is not given automatic custody, visitation rights, or other legal access to the child once paternity has been established and child support is collected. It is a state whose laws will deem a child abandoned in the event that a parent does not have contact with a child for a certain amount of time.

A single mother-friendly political climate is one in which the current elected leaders do not regard women, single women, or single mothers as being responsible for crime, poverty, or other social challenges. Single mother-friendly legal and social climates normally have a focus on charity and public and health resources. Race relations are often positive and dynamic in these social climates. "Blue states" are often more mother-friendly, but not always. Whether a social climate is hostile is often indicated by the level of extremism in political views rather than whether the popular view is conservative or liberal.

A single mother-to-be will often know right away when her social climate is single mother-hostile. Abortion and adoption are often main topics in these hostile environments, and there is a denial of the importance of separation of church and state. Race relations are often contentious and oppositional in single mother-hostile environments, as people who see themselves in various social groups feel they need to huddle together like musk oxen in order to defend themselves against the opposition of their values. In a single mother-hostile environment, women's rights are often swept under the carpet or mocked. There is often religious fundamentalism and ample discussion of God in politics and in schools, and the blocking of scientific information.

The following child support discussion begins assuming that your social and political climate is either neutral on the mother-friendly side. We will tackle discussing the mother-hostile issues later. But on order to get a well-rounded education on these issues, I am going to hope that you read the entire section, whether or not you think it will affect you, as there are always potential positive and negative climate aspects you will encounter no matter where you live.

Child Support
Although our government makes a rare exhibition of wisdom with its implementation of child support enforcement, our *society* works hard to guarantee that she who ventures to obtain child support will not do so without having to endure a certain amount of shame. This is one instance in which certain members of our society judge others to their own detriment. After all, if the government can force deadbeat fathers to pay a 20 percent pittance of their income to help raise their own children, won't that take the financial burden off other government assistance programs (welfare, for example) whose effectiveness is constantly being questioned? How anyone feels justified in judging someone who goes to the root of a problem to find its solution is way beyond me, but you see a lot of this kind of hypocrisy when you've endured single pregnancy with your eyes open!

I do understand the wide diversity of circumstances that single mothers-to-be can find themselves in. It is without judgment that I will express one of the few imperatives within this book: If a man has anything whatsoever to do with his child as a father—whether paternity is confirmed or simply accepted, if the father has custody or visitation or not—if the man claims that he is the father of the child, child support needs to come with that status.

Keep in mind that this is also true in the reverse—if the father is the most appropriate caretaker for the child, it is the mother who should pay the child support. The child's needs should be at least partially supported by the non-custodial parent. In most single pregnancy scenarios, the custodial parent will be the mother. There are exceptions to the mother being the child support recipient—sometimes they are through an agreement of both parties (the mother travels extensively for work and the father has a stable home and a consistent routine), some of them are the result of bad court outcomes (the father has successfully convinced the judge that the mother is unfit), and some are the result of appropriate court outcomes (the mother is indeed unfit due to drugs, crime, abuse, etc.). Simply stated, if one parent is taking care of the majority of the child's needs, the other parent needs to contribute—and in single pregnancy situations, the parent most often caring for the majority of the child's needs is the mother.

Although there is a widespread and popular belief in our society (often bolstered by gossip slathered upon a weak-minded audience) that those women who wind up in unexpected pregnancies have done so with an intention to "victimize" the unborn child's father, "trap" him in an unwanted marriage, and "get money" if he doesn't cooperate. However, the unfortunate truth is that the biggest victims in this strange belief and the effects of its popularity are not the fathers but are indeed the children—and in one way or another, we all pick up the tab for children in poverty.

Interestingly, despite the popularity of the "money hungry single mother" stereotype, it appears that in the majority of cases, the pressure for single pregnant women to prove noble intentions is much stronger than the desire for food and earthly possessions. According to the surveys filled out by single pregnant women who have participated in an ongoing non-scientific poll on my web site, most uninsured single pregnant women who make between $24,000 and $35,000 annually (too much to qualify for Medicaid but too little to live comfortably with medical bills associated with pregnancy and childbirth) do not plan to seek child support. The most popular reason: They don't want to force involvement of the child's father in the child's life. Sadly, these women and their children not only deserve child support—many of them also need it.

In order to identify the reasons for obtaining child support, I must first discuss the myths associated with getting child support, and preface these myths with an opinion developed after my having fought a lengthy and expensive court battle that ate up practically all of the back child support that was granted when the hearing was over: The best way to obtain child support is not to go through an attorney and the court system, but is instead to take advantage of the free services offered by the Child Support Enforcement Division (CSED) (also sometimes called Child Support Services Division, CSSD). I feel that CSED is a more effective medium for obtaining child support because 1) it's a free service provided by our Federal Government, 2) Unlike a court battle, CSED does not allow the opposition time to prepare a counter argument, and 3) the people at CSED are accustomed to dealing with single pregnancy, whereas family attorneys mostly deal with child custody and visitation issues as a result of a divorce.

Some will argue that going to court takes less time. This is simply not true. When I sought a child support and custody agreement through court, I didn't get my settlement until a year and a half after my son was born, whereas a friend who went through CSED got her first payment within a few short months. The fact is, if you are organized, diligent, stable, live in a legal that's generally mother-friendly, and your child's father is not a combative or vengeful person, your experience with CSED will almost certainly have the same results as a court battle without costing you a penny.

Things to consider:
Child Support from a Resistant Father
In the event that the child's father has made himself scarce throughout a woman's pregnancy, it is often possible for the mother to prove that this man has no business being in the child's life. In the event that the child's father has been violent, unstable, cruel, manipulative, destructive, or seems to have improper motives, it is likewise possible to keep him away from the child if indeed the events were documented (always document phone calls, messages, conversations, quotes, etcetera in your interactions with him and keep them in a file or day planner. Do not throw old day planners away. File them instead). A great way to document interactions is to insist that all your communication be in the form of e-mail, and save or print the e-mails. This may be painful at times, but if your child's father has been unreasonable, insulting, uses profanity or abusive language, or refuses to cooperate with you, it will show in his e-mails. If this is the way you plan to do things, you must refrain from doing anything that makes you seem unreasonable as well, even though you may very well have been antagonized to the point of wanting to explode. If comments are made about things you've done in the past, your "reputation," or any other personal comments, rest assured that your actions are probably going to be of little interest to any authority, so do not dignify them with a response—let it go, and respond calmly as though the comments had never been made. Also, make sure you are not emotionally manipulated into "steering away from the point" of your correspondence. Ask only what is necessary, and respond only to what is necessary (read **Chapter 7** before initiating or continuing correspondence with the baby's father). If your child's father lobs personal attacks at you, keep your cool, and don't strike back with a "what about what *you* did?" If lack of cooperation is not documented, the mother can still often win anyone over through cooperation, honesty, and exhibiting stable conduct—but documentation does indeed help.

I know of one case in which a single woman with a baby went after child support from the baby's natural father, who had since married another woman. He tried at length to convince the counselors that the baby should live with him and his new wife, doing his best to ruin the reputation of the baby's mother. In the end, he had to pay child support, was not allowed visitation, and all he got out of the deal was a photograph of the baby.

Visiting a counselor at the CSED *can* be a potentially humiliating experience. People who work in this field are individuals, and have their own judgments about your situation. You could be asked again and again whether you're sure of the child's paternity, which can take anyone to the emotional breaking point, especially when there's already been a lot of denial in the baby-father's camp. But if that's the case, think of the counselor as though she were a judge. She sees so many sad and hopeless situations that she may assume the worst about you when you step into her office. Take it upon yourself to prove her wrong. Heroes are those who change people's minds. Pave the way for all of the single pregnant women who will come after you. Show this person that stable, kind, and worthy single mothers-to-be are the norm rather than the exception.

Paternity:

Paternity is certainly one of the more sensitive issues when trying to obtain child support, but establishing paternity may not be as hard as you might think. The easiest way to establish paternity is for the father of your child to sign a paternity affidavit while you are still pregnant. If your child's father has an interest in having a workable relationship with you and the child, he may be willing to do this much. In the event that your child's father will sign a paternity affidavit, there is a chance that the two of you can eventually have an acceptable visitation arrangement, and may even be effective co-parents. However, more often than not, the child's father wants to run far and fast from any responsibility, denying that there is any chance that this child is his until he has proof. If your child's father is denying paternity, it is safest to wait until the child is born to have a paternity test. If your child's father is employed, the CSED will authorize a paternity test, which he will often have to pay for. However, if it is not his child, you will likely end up having to pay for the paternity test yourself. If paternity is established, the wages of your child's father will be garnished, and you will receive about 20 percent of his monthly income.

Sometimes the mother will be granted "back child support" for medical expenses and the time she spent pregnant, and sometimes she won't. But as I said before, the cost of my court battle was just about equal to half of my medical expenses, so try to see your glass as half full rather than half empty if you don't get all you were hoping for.

Another aspect of establishing paternity that must be noted: *Do not claim to be certain of a child's paternity if you are not 100 percent certain!* If there is more than one possibility, do not blame yourself or feel ashamed, but do not bring any undue attention upon yourself by claiming that a certain individual is your child's father. Probably the best way to protect yourself from judgment is to counter any questions with "I am keeping the identity of my child's father a secret." If you are on speaking terms with the person you believe to be your child's father, he will likely be more cooperative with you if you let him know that you are not publicizing his potential involvement, and that you'd like to legally confirm his paternity before assuming that he is indeed the baby's father. Doing so will allow him to choose whether or not he wants to be involved as more than the payer of child support, and in many cases may keep you out of harm's way.

Will my seeking Child Support Negatively Affect my Child?

Although certain members of our society (often consisting of deadbeat parents and the people who love them) would like us to believe that collecting child support will be humiliating for our children, this is simply not true.

First of all, many children are from single parent homes, and many others are living within extremely dysfunctional two-parent families. Half of all marriages end in divorce and many of those marriages have produced children. Although it is not necessarily a good thing, these broken homes have become the norm. Although your circumstances are different from those of divorced women, the result is the same: Single parent household. Thankfully, because single parent homes have become the norm, coming from a single parent home is no longer an effective vehicle for people to ostracize or shame children.

Can You Spend it on Yourself?

Please don't buy into the idea that any child support you spend on yourself has been "squandered." If your child is housed, fed, clothed, and protected, you are doing your job as a mom. If you can take care of all your child's basic needs on your income alone, lucky you! But does that mean it is somehow correct for you to turn down child support? Heck no!

If you need a better pair of shoes in order to have a better day at work, buy them. Besides, until your child is in kindergarten, it is likely that you won't have any child support left over to spend after day care is paid for. True, it would not be taking the high road to use your child support for nicer shoes in the event that your child's needs are not met, but *your* needs are extremely important too. You are the one who holds everything up. Let your child's level of happiness and wellbeing speak of your integrity.

Reasons you should Consider Yourself Entitled to Child Support:
Reason #1: Accountability belongs with the accountable!

Regardless of the circumstances that led to your pregnancy, you did not fertilize yourself. Although our society loves to accuse single pregnant women of scheming, planning, and trapping, you are no guiltier of taking advantage of someone than is the child's father. After all, was he so dense that he was unaware of the fact that the core purpose of sexual intercourse is reproduction? Yes, it is a pleasurable activity, and the media like to perpetuate the idea that it is a pastime free of consequence for its participants, but any doofus knows that nothing short of removing one's reproductive organs is 100 percent effective in preventing pregnancy, which is why most people don't bother with feeding birth control pills to our cats and dogs. Although it is no laughing matter—because apparently it does happen every once in a while—ask yourself this question: Did you *force* the father of your child to have sex with you? If the answer is "no," then you are no more responsible for the outcome of your pregnancy than he is.

Some people will say that this is not a valid argument because our country provides you with a choice as to whether or not to have your baby. But based on your personal or religious beliefs, you truly might not have a choice in the matter. And if you are Pro-Choice, do you *have* to exercise your right to terminate a pregnancy simply because all contributing parties do not agree that you should have your child? Heck no! You don't need to exercise every right you support. You're taking responsibility, and you had a very short window within which to make your decision. Is *he* taking ownership in his part in this? Even if he is 100 percent involved, he will have far less to do than *you* will.

And although certain men like to yell and scream about the fact that they're getting 20 percent of their income taken away, the sacrifices you are soon to make are likely to be much greater. When you combine the physical and economic challenges of pregnancy and parenthood with the fact that working women still make only three-fourths of a man's income, I *hardly* think that a lousy few hundred dollars a month will adequately compensate you.

Furthermore, babies are expensive. Who *should* pay for your child's needs? Although lots of people fall on hard times at certain points in their lives and have no choice but to take advantage of government assistance, do your best to use government assistance as a last resort. You don't want to be a part of the government spending problem; you want to be a part of the personal accountability *solution*. If it is at all possible (and in most cases with Child Support it *is* possible), go to the *source* of the problem to find its solution. After all, *you are* going to be personally accountable, so should he be.

Reason #2: Your child might end up with better medical insurance!
In the event that your child's father has health insurance through his job and you don't, guess what! He may have to add your child to his insurance policy. You may think that you can handle the expense of occasional well baby visits and those vaccinations you choose to put your faith in, but in the event that your child develops a problem, having your child on his father's health insurance might save the life of your child, and might save you from financial ruin.

When my son was two years old, I had a very frightening incident when he took a bite out of a cashew, and his face instantly swelled up and turned red. Although my doctor might have been trying to quell my panic when he reacted calmly to our crisis, my next step was to see an allergy specialist, which would have cost me more than a thousand dollars. If not for my son's father's insurance, it would have been a financial impossibility.

The allergist's findings were significant: My son had anaphylaxis to cashews, peanuts, and a strong allergy to cats. If my son had swallowed that cashew, he may have died. If my son had eaten a piece of Halloween candy with peanuts in it, he may have died. Although cat hair didn't seem to bother him, if my son had ever been severely bitten by my cat (who thereafter lived at my parents' house and was put in the garage when my son came over), he may have died as a result. In the event that I hadn't had the financial freedom to find out whether or not the cashew incident was something to worry about, I might have found out about my son's allergies the hard way, through an unexpected and untimely death!

You may be surprised at who has health insurance and who doesn't. Even certain fast food restaurants have health insurance policies for their employees. Although in some states, people living below the poverty income level will have the opportunity to get medical care for free or on a sliding scale based on their income, many women will find no such luck. Your child's father may not want you to know whether or not he has health insurance, but if he does, the CSED will find out.

Reason #3: Every little bit helps
Consider these four scenarios:

You have found a great, professional, dedicated, full-time multilingual babysitter whom you really like and trust, and she only lives one block away from you, which would eliminate an hour of subway scrambling in your morning routine, but she costs two hundred dollars more than your other option. You could really use an extra hour of sleep in the morning, as well as an extra hour to unwind in the evening, but after food, rent, and utility bills, you only have two hundred dollars in the bank and that's cutting it way too close.

Your child has been humming the alphabet song since before she could say "mama." Recently, you heard her sounding it out on her xylophone. You know you have a virtuoso on your hands, but you don't have any formal training in music, and music lessons cost eighty dollars a month. After your expenses, you only have fifty dollars left in your bank account.

You have an opportunity to interview for the job of your dreams, but this company has a professional dress code, and you don't have any dress shoes because you've been delivering pizzas for the last two years. You are well qualified for this position and know you can get it, but you don't have a credit card, and you don't have the money in your account to get the appropriate shoes to make the right impression for this job.

You've educated yourself on food safety issues, and you have decided that you only want to feed your child organic vegetables and meat from livestock that has never been fed antibiotics, but if you do that, your normal grocery bill increases by twenty dollars a week.

You have a right and an obligation to make the right choices in order to provide a better life for yourself and your child, but if the money is not there, it's not there. This list of scenarios can go on and on, but to bring it all home, I'll ask you this: Would two hundred dollars a month help?

In the event that you do get child support, it will most likely be more than two hundred dollars a month. If that can make a difference in your quality of life, you should embrace the opportunity to make a better life for yourselves.

Even if your bills are all covered by your own income, don't feel bad about getting this little bit more. If you are able to save it for the child, then do that. When you're flying on an airplane, what is it that they tell you about the oxygen masks? Put the mask on yourself before you help anyone else (including children) with it. You won't be much help to anyone if you pass out from oxygen deprivation before you get that mask on your child. If you are feeling deprived and depressed, it is likely that you are not going to be the best advocate for your child's advancement.

Reason #4: *A good mother knows better than to let pride stand in her way of making a decision that benefits herself and her baby.*

Pride is a confusing characteristic. It can be a virtue when it helps us to stand tall against what we know is wrong, but when a person's pride isn't kept in check, it can prevent us from seeing what needs to be done in order to survive. Let's look back to **Chapter 4**, when I told the story about my ex-fiancé who was humiliated by my habit of picking coins up off the street. He didn't like people perceiving that we might be of a lower class—and in his mind, this humiliation took precedence over the fact that we were in fact hungry. Until he made his feelings known to me, I didn't realize that my habit of collecting pennies would negatively affect him, and after his feelings were explained, they still didn't make much sense.

This brings about an important question: How was it that the intangible quality of pride could be more painful to my ex-fiancé than physical hunger was to me?

Answer: He was an insecure, selfish asshole. His pride, along with the image he wanted to project to the world, was more important than my hunger.

Now don't get me wrong, not everyone who does things out of pride is an insecure, selfish asshole. It just so happens that some of the most capable and honest single pregnant women choose not to seek child support because they want to show the world that their choices to keep their children were not caused by an intention to coerce a man into marriage or get his money, and the pressure to prove this to society is aggrandized by our society's negative and judgmental reaction to unsupported pregnancies. This strategy works well if you're a millionaire like Elizabeth Hurley, and we can all appreciate her comment that billionaire "baby daddy" Steven Bing's child support was "not wanted and not welcome" after he had publicly denied paternity of her son later to be proven wrong (surprise, surprise! Oh, wait—I wasn't too surprised, and I don't think she was either). But she has the means to give herself and son everything they need to thrive. In the event that you make any less than seventy thousand dollars a year (maybe more, depending on where you live), guess what? It's not likely that you're going to have extra child support money lying around.

Yes, people can be cruel. No, many people don't understand. Yes, some insecure and unhappy people would love a reason to gossip about you and put themselves above you. Yes, your child's father may relish the opportunity to tell his loser friends that you tried to trap him into a marriage and that you're after his money. Yes, there may be a whole crowd of people who will feel some sort of triumph when they feel they can comment negatively on your character based on their little knowledge of and bizarre opinions about your situation.

Ladies, these people are idiots. They may even be the majority, but they are still idiots. You should not worry about what they think of you. Do you like *them*? I don't! And guess what? What goes around comes around. They'll get their turn, and by that time, you will be well on your way and will have more important things to do than to triumph over their misfortune. The only person who can make or break you is YOU, not them. As human beings, we do depend on public opinion for our survival to a certain extent, but rather than worrying about protecting yourself from the judgments of the ignorant, worry about impressing your supervisor at work, your true friends and family who care about you unconditionally, and your child.

Remember that *you have nothing to prove!* If you know that you did not wind up pregnant to trap some guy, why do you need to waste your precious time proving that to people who will not like you one way or the other? And if *even if you did*, oh well! You didn't do it on your own. Moving on! As a single mother-to-be, you are already a maverick. You have already proven that you can go against society's expectations and stand alone when there's no one worthy of standing beside you. Don't let your pride or your fear of idiot mob mentality keep you from getting the funds that *even the government* understands you are entitled to in order to effectively bring up your child.

If after reading this you are still not planning to seek child support, then listen to your own heart and mind about this situation, as there are thousands of circumstances that can affect your decision that go beyond the scope of what was discussed in this chapter.

You probably still have a few months to think about whether or not to seek child support, so just make the best decision you can in order to protect yourself and your child.

Child Support and Custody in a Mother-Hostile Social Climate
In my opinion, a mother-hostile legal climate is one where elected judges grant custody or unsupervised visitation rights to a child's natural father who has been consistently absent, physically or emotionally abusive, destructive, or has a criminal record; and where impoverished or minority people are blamed by politicians and the community at large for crime, unemployment, and other social issues. Some judges will grant unsupervised visitation or even custody to fathers simply because the babies' mothers have sought child support. It should also be mentioned that some judges, regardless of where they are, consistently "reward" unwitting fathers with rights they did not earn simply because they show initiative in wanting to be involved, not understanding that involvement is often simply to seek vengeance on the child's mother and minimize child support. This is a chapter section in which the lines between child support and custody get extremely blurred, as they are so intermingled.

You may be surprised to learn which states have mother-hostile laws, as I was shocked to hear the story of a reader who had to leave Colorado to give birth to her child to prevent that child's father from literally taking the baby away from her (it should be noted that similar threats are often lobbed and rarely followed up on—it is simply an issue of intimidation and control, which equates to emotional abuse of the mother and baby, and absolutely *should* prevent a father from gaining custodial rights).

As I said before, men who pelt threats of taking a child away are usually just blowing off steam and have no idea how and would never *want* to take care of a baby, but are instead simply interested in abusing *the child's mother*. In addition, causing stress for a pregnant woman is abusive to the child inside her, as the child will feel the stress, even if it can't process exactly what's going on. But many men in our society have been taught that it is their right to behave in such a way. In my opinion, this is just plain wrong, but not everybody sees it this way.

Question: My state has mother-hostile legal and social climate. I have done my research, and have concluded that I am not going to seek child support because of how it may compromise my custody rights, and believe that my child's father can and will take my baby away. What can I do to protect myself and my baby?

Answer: Diffuse the energy: Sometimes a woman can gain control over this situation by simply acting as though (and believing that) the threat doesn't exist, and refusing to engage her energy into the argument, refusing to feed this man's power with her fear. A man would have to have a lot of energy, dedication, follow-through, and sometimes a lot of money in order to take a baby away from a mother, and if he's not getting any energy from you, he will likely eventually run out of interest in continuing the drama.

Cut off all contact with the child's natural father: If your child's father is in the same social scene that you're in, this might be easier said than done, but I recommend cutting off all contact with any "natural father" who has been anything other than kind, supportive, and cooperative. Sometimes people assume that abandoned contact with the child's father is an admission of guilt that there was dishonesty in the paternity "accusation." The clear drawback in this situation is that it may disrupt your social circle, and some people will feel that you were just part of a grand manipulative scheme. This has potential to hurt your pride and break your heart. You may even need to find a whole new group of friends, and may have to seek emotional healing for the trauma caused by this situation. The bonus, however, is that when a man assumes that the baby is not his, he will often leave you alone and let you get about your business.

Prepare your argument: Following are a few things that courts often consider when it comes to child custody cases. In some cases, you can maintain your sole physical and legal custody of the child while getting child support even if you live in a state with mother-hostile laws. In the event that you are ever required to appear before anyone regarding the care of your child, your having performed the following tasks will help identify you as the child's primary caretaker:

- Feeding the infant
- Feeding younger children
- Changing diapers
- Holding/cuddling/comforting the baby or child
- Preparing meals/ researching nutrition
- Grocery shopping
- Taking initiative with medical care
- Taking initiative with parenting choices
- Dressing
- Doing laundry
- Buying clothes
- Bathing/washing hair/styling hair/ haircuts
- Brushing teeth
- Putting the child to bed
- Observing a regular feeding and sleeping schedule
- Researching school/day care transportation & tuition costs
- Care of sick child
- Cleaning the home
- Maintaining the home

Like I said, most combative and drama-addicted men don't know the first thing about doing these things. Whatever you do, do not share this list with your child's father as an outline for your expectations unless you have a completely peaceful, respectful, and cooperative relationship or—if not peaceful—one that has already been enforced by the courts.

Move to another state: It may sound extreme, but if you and your child's father are going to be engaging in a long-term battle for rights, your best bet may be to move from the state in which you are currently living to give birth to your baby, and possibly to stay. If you have family or close friends living in another state with child support and custody laws that are more "mother-friendly" *or* if you simply need to hide from a frightening baby daddy who is hellbent against letting you love peacefully, talk to them about possibly moving to their town. Assure them (and yourself) that you are not going to bring any of this drama with you—that you are making a clean break. If you are currently living in the same town as (and depend on) your parents, see if they are willing to move with you. Depending on your relationship with your family, you may be surprised to find that they are perfectly willing to make a fresh start with you (my own family was gearing up to do exactly that, but we eventually decided against it). In some cases (again, it depends entirely on the state in which you give birth and the state in which your child's father lives), you can seek child support from a safe distance without ever having to worry about your custodial rights being compromised.

At the time of this writing, you can access the Federal Child Support Enforcement site at www.acf.hhs.gov/programs/cse. From this page you can access the links to the state pages, find your state, and get the information you need.

If the Cat Comes Back After the Storm is Over

Although I often highly recommend doing whatever you can to get child support, I just as often warn against giving up any of your rights as the custodial parent of your child. Sometimes a formerly absent father will come back onto the scene after a year or two and expect to be welcomed into the child's life. Sometimes this works out just fine, especially in the event that he is willing to pay back child support and has made positive strides in his life. However, even if he has cleaned up his act, if you have healed from what he put you through, and if it seems reasonable to allow this father into his child's life, you must still exercise caution.

We've all had hardships. As one who is surviving single pregnancy, you may feel that you've shouldered your share of hardship for a while. I too felt this way when my son's father decided he wanted to be a part of my son's life. I thought it would be a relief to have someone help me with the responsibilities of raising my son. I thought that my son's father's family would realize the error of their ways when they found that I hadn't been lying about my son's paternity, and I figured that just because he denied paternity didn't necessarily mean that he would be a bad parent. When I took my son's father to court for child support, I also allowed him to have partial custody.

As mentioned before, one year later it was found that my son had dangerous allergies to peanuts, cashews, pistachios, cats, and a mild allergy to dogs (which has since subsided) that might trigger his asthma. Although it was heartbreaking, I got rid of my cat, and stopped having peanuts and cashews in my home. As incidents of dangerous reactions to peanuts and cashews were becoming commonplace, many of the treats I would give my son began carrying labels that warned of possible peanut contamination. Per the doctor's orders I read labels each and every time, and one by one, practically every candy bar at the supermarket was deemed dangerous for my son to eat.

When my son came home from his father's house, I would often find M&Ms and Milky Way bars in my son's pockets. I would ask my son about it and he would say that his father said they were okay because they didn't have peanuts in them, although the label clearly stated "may contain traces of peanuts and tree nuts."

To make a long story short, the next two years provided several similar incidents. Every time I would talk to my son's father, and every time he would assure me that he was reading the labels. At about the fifteenth incident, my son's father said, "Well, nothing has happened yet, so I'm going to continue to give him whatever I want to give him." At that time, I took him to court to sue for full custody. It should be noted that during the same verbal exchange, I had said "I'm starting to think that you may be *trying* to kill my son!" No, my point was not taken. This comment came back to haunt me again and again, and much of my time, energy, and money was dedicated to proving that I was not "insane." Let this be your lesson not to allow your emotions to get the best of you when speaking about important things to your child's father.

Five months and four thousand dollars later, my son's father finally agreed not to give our son candy bars that may contain traces of peanuts and tree nuts. I was granted several court orders to help insure that my son's father would more properly observe my son's allergies, but because we had already been co-parenting for two years "without incident" (although I felt that there had been several "incidents" that demonstrated my son's father's inability to adequately parent), not only I was not granted full custody, but my son's father was given even more time, and my child support was reduced to almost nothing! Then my son's father moved in with his girlfriend who had an indoor dog, although my son was still allergic to dogs. I'll assume you get the point about my eventual loss of control and I'll stop here.

This would never have had a chance to happen if I hadn't given my son's father the benefit of the doubt. Forgiveness is a good thing, but my son's father (and his family) had never even acknowledged their trespasses, and had never *asked* for forgiveness—to this day, they feel that they have done nothing wrong. Remember that you can forgive a person through your heart and let the anger go without giving up any of your control in the physical world.

Yes, giving my son's father any rights whatsoever was the biggest mistake in my life so far, as once a parent has custodial rights, it is nearly impossible to take them away. Please learn from my mistakes: No matter how hard life seems, do not give up any custody of your child! Worrying for your child's safety is never worth free child care.

Yes, some people have successfully managed to have a peaceful arrangement with their child's fathers, but don't take for granted that this is going to happen even if he seems like a good person. A friend of mine has a great relationship worked out with her daughter's father: She has sole legal and physical custody of her child, and her child's father has full visitation (the right to see the child, etc.). If she ever wanted to move away, there would be nothing standing in her way. If she wanted her child to have an all-organic diet or to decide against certain potentially dangerous vaccinations, her child's father would have to respect her wishes. As one who is a kind and respectful person who simply wants a relationship with his child, her child's father is happy with this arrangement.

◆ ◆ ◆

Although some women experience maternal instincts sooner than others, once we become mothers, most of us become acutely aware of (and take action against) any compromise of our child's safety. If you put yourself in the position to worry regularly, you pose a significant risk to both your physical and mental health, and new single mothers have enough challenges to their sanity—they do not need to throw another risk factor on the heap! If your child's father wants to come back into your lives, he needs to do his part to bolster your survival. You may decide to let him have visitation, but please don't let him have any right to undermine your well thought-out decisions or potentially harm your child. Instead, hire a real babysitter: One who knows that *you* are the boss.

Chapter Seven

Communication with the Baby's Father

Ideally, both the mother and natural father of baby—if not married or otherwise partnered—will communicate in a mutually respectful way in order to facilitate a viable co-parenting relationship. However, as many former single mothers-to-be, single mothers, and even single fathers will tell you, there are situations in which this is realistic, and situations in which it is not—and there is no one-size-fits-all rule that covers every possible scenario a single pregnant woman might face.

When there is a question of paternity, an out-and-out paternity denial, abandonment of a planned pregnancy, an unresolved injustice, or simply a struggle for control, communication with your child's father can be abusive, contentious, or simply ineffective. In many dangerous situations mentioned in previous chapters, particularly those in which the mother cannot depend on the law catching up with one's actions, the mother-to-be may decide that she is going to completely cut off communication with her child's father (we will discuss how to do this later in this chapter).

In other situations, she may feel that it is important to give the baby's father the opportunity to evolve in order to one day have a relationship with the child and—possibly—an effective co-parenting relationship with the mother. However, a fact that has been proven to me time and time again through my advocacy work is this: The only way this can be accomplished is to for the mother to conduct herself with the utmost integrity and self-respect, and to refuse to engage in communication that does not meet her in this high place. This is particularly important if the father has been insulting, emotionally abusive, or avoidant.

YOU Set the Tone

Rest assured that when communication has been bad, healing is still possible. However, more often than not, a mother interested in co-parenting accepts certain potentially damaging lifestyle and communication traits in order to empower a relationship between the father and the child, and ends up stuck navigating those qualities for the duration of the child's life as a minor (and possibly beyond). The important thing to remember is this: Do not stoop to meet him on a low level, and do not make compromises in order to foster this relationship—instead, insist that he rise to meet you at a level of high integrity and functionality.

Some people will say to a mother in this situation that dealing with an angry, abusive, or avoidant man is her "penance," that this is "what (she's) gotten (herself) into." This, of course is an antiquated cultural tenet that is quite the opposite of the truth: To accept this type of treatment is to accept abuse. It is more accurate to say that it is a mother's obligation to herself and her child NOT to take it.

If your conversations with your child's father have typically degraded into insults, accusations, and cutting remarks, there is only one thing you can do: require that all communication be in writing, and ideally to have it sent to an e-mail that is not your primary email, if possible (an email account that you will not have to look at every day for work, bills, or your social life). Nothing can screw up a productive day at work, a peaceful night of sleep, or a positive outlook on your day like feeling that you need to defend yourself by responding to a nasty-gram, especially when you are likely to already be physically, mentally, and emotionally exhausted. You need to be able to deal with it only when you have the time and the energy, and—if possible—in the company of a trusted and non-reactive friend, relative, or advocate who can commit to momentarily disengaging her emotions and objectively reading the email in order to tell you whether there is anything in it that truly needs a response from you. As one who will be pregnant for months, know that it is your right to take all the time you need to respond to communication.

Of course, having everything in writing means that you too will have to exercise self-control. Remember that if these emails are read by a judge, you will only come out smelling like roses if you refrain from engaging in any drama or making any counter-threats. If you don't exercise control in your written communication, regardless of what the truth is, your baby's father might have some evidence that you are seeking revenge rather than doing what's best for the baby. Although you may have counter-evidence, to play this game will simply result in long, costly, and stressful litigation. Unless you are laying down rules and expectations (which might take more than a few words), keep your emails short and to-the-point, and only say what is absolutely necessary.

Through my work with single mothers-to-be, I have many times been the wing-woman in this scenario, and I have seen the same things come up again and again, including paternity denial, threats to "take the baby away," and even professions of love—sometimes all in the same sentence! On the other hand, I have seen honest attempts at functional communication that were rejected due to lingering anger over unresolved injustices. Always give yourself time to heal from anger before you engage in any regular communication. Blowing up, although natural, is looked down upon by authorities.

Following are two examples: A message that should be ignored, and one that shows an honest attempt at communication. This first message is an example of something that should be documented (printed up or safely electronically filed), but is not an honest and respectful attempt at communication:

> *What's up? I was just thinking about you and the baby, and I am really hoping that you will do the smart thing and just come talk to me. I really want to be there for the birth, and I've been told it's my right to be there and to know when you are going to the hospital because this is my baby too, and I expect to be in the delivery room for the birth of my own child. You act like it's all about you. It's not like I haven't seen it all before, so I can't help but to wonder as to why you think that's not a good idea! After I talked to Dave and the guys, and they told me how you acted at that party back in October, I've got to ask myself if this could really be my baby anyway. Is that it? Is there going to be another guy there? Because if there is, you know I can bring Katie too and it will all be cool, although I know you are still bitter about her. You might as well accept that she's going to be our baby's family too. Anyway, I talked to an attorney, and he says that I can get 50/50 custody right off the bat, but I'm thinking, wouldn't it be best for the baby to be in a two-parent family? I just want to get your take on that, because Katie is willing to step in to make that happen. So call me. We really need to hash this out like adults, okay? You can't keep avoiding me and running from this. Just set aside your bitterness and do what's right for the child, okay?*

Yes, this is horrible. And yet—it's rather common. The point of this communication is not to make any ground, but is instead to attack the mother's self-esteem and insult her in hopes that she will submit and surrender her control over the situation. Despite the fact that this is sure to be a bad memory, this e-mail needs to be printed up or otherwise saved.

When I've seen e-mails such as these sent to me by single mothers-to-be, if I didn't respond to my counselee in time, sometimes I'd read a return e-mail that took hours to compose, responding to each and every one of the father's points as though they were valid concerns rather than simple attacks. Know for certain that an e-mail like this is not about the baby or the situation—it's about you.

Let's take a closer look at it:

"What's up?" Although using this type of language is a relatively minor offense, this is downplaying the seriousness and formality of the situation.

"Do the smart thing..." This is not only an insult to your intelligence, but is also a threat. It implies that to make a choice other than that which is dictated will have negative consequences for you.

"Come talk to me..." Asking you to engage in conversation where there are no witnesses rather than saying what he needs to say in writing, where potential threats and misbehavior will not be a matter of your word against his.

"It's my right to be there..." Indicating that your privacy, safety, body, and peace of mind were forfeited when you engaged in sexual relations with him, and that the child is his property. This comment is meant to make you feel ashamed.

"Talked to Dave and the guys..." This is trying to make you feel disliked or outnumbered—especially by men—and engage you in defending your reputation and integrity (this is something no man with honest intentions would want for the mother of his child to have to do).

"Katie could be there..." This is another patriarchal tenet that his current woman is an extension of him, and outranks you in his life as one who is currently "approved of," so she also has a right to invade your privacy in matters regarding his assumed "property," the child and the body you forfeited when you had sexual relations.

"I talked to an attorney..." This is another threat. And rest assured, any attorney that would claim that the father could get 50/50 right off the bat knows that a fool and his money are soon parted (bear in mind that although there are exceptions, a woman who is not currently engaged in criminal activity often has little to worry about in terms of losing her child or even compromising in custody—unless she engages in too much unproductive documented debate). In the vast majority of cases, a man who makes this claim has not in fact talked to any attorney at all, but wants you to think he has.

"Like adults..." This is indicating that your behavior is childlike rather than protective of yourself and the baby.

"You can't..." Commenting on what he thinks your rights or abilities are.

"Your bitterness..." This is indicating that your refusal to engage in his desired mode of communication and yield to his requests is because you still want him, something many women will engage their valuable energy into disproving.

Understand that there is nothing in this communication that needs to be responded to—and please do not respond. This is a collection of disrespectful threats and insults, meant only to knock you off your game.

Now let's take a look at how the same requests can be made respectfully:

I have been thinking about you and the baby, and I hope you will choose to talk to me. I would like to be notified when you are going into labor, and I hope you will give me the opportunity to see the baby when he is born, and that you will let me know if there's anything I can bring to help you to help out. For legal reasons, I would like a paternity test. Since there is no question in your mind regarding paternity, I understand that it is my responsibility to pay for it. This is not in any way an indication that I don't believe you, but is a standard legal procedure for your protection as well as mine. I want to be an active and consistent part of this child's life, and want to assure you that any partner I have in my life will understand and respect that you are this child's mother, and will respect my intention to have a civil and productive co-parenting relationship with you. Please let me know what I can do to help us achieve this.

Before you cringe, know that I have seen emails like this one too. If the father of your baby is not a criminal, an addict not in recovery, an abuser, and is not one who has been traditionally foul in his communication, this does show enough maturity and desire for cooperation to indicate that a co-parenting relationship might be feasible. Also bear in mind that a person who speaks like this just may have done some real research, which might have included talking to an attorney, but seems to have gotten the right advice: "You are going to have to work with this woman for the rest of your life. You need to take responsibility for your part of it so this does not turn into an 18+ year mess."

Although many women are emotionally triggered by the mention of a paternity test, by now you probably know that it is standard procedure for any pregnancy in which the couple was not cohabitating or where there was the possibility of infidelity on either person's part, and should also be a condition imposed on a man who eventually wants any rights at all in the child's future. Although you may need some time to heal from your relationship, especially if the baby's father was guilty of the infidelity or another breach of relationship agreement, being civil is something you are going to eventually have to roll with. Also remember this: Cooperation and trust are two different things. Later in this chapter I will demonstrate why it is important to appreciate and reciprocate cooperation, but not to trust that it will last.

If your child's father is not a dangerous person but has some character flaws (lying, cheating, cowardice, laziness, leaving the relationship when the pregnancy was announced, etc.) and you still feel that it is best that he be in the child's life, you may be able to heal from whatever injustices occurred by remembering this: If you are willing to settle for liar, cheater, or a run-from-the-hard-times person in a romantic relationship, then that's all you will ever get. People deserve better than this, so insist upon better for your future romantic relationships.

Naturally, you may need time to recover from such things in order to even the playing field and move forward. Think hard about what you need: willing reimbursement for half (or more, depending on your incomes) of your maternity and labor/ delivery costs, for example. A legally filed co-parenting agreement that shared custody could be achieved after three years of consistent support in the event that the child's father remains local, accessible, cooperative, and out of legal trouble. That your child's father show up on time to every scheduled visitation and compensate you if he does not. Any man who wants to play fair will be willing to do this much. If this is what you ask and he balks, you know your answer: Co-parenting is not going to work out well, at least not until he realizes what it means to be fair.

If the father of your baby is willing to play fair, there are some incentives to committing yourself to healing with the intention of having smooth relations. It is more likely that you will attract calm, cooperative, baggage-free partners in your future if you exhibit this behavior yourself. Of course, being able to exhibit this behavior will depend on how well you have enforced your boundaries over what you will accept—and it is neither necessary nor recommended that you martyr yourself and tolerate abuse or economic ruin in order to include your child's father in his or her life.

Let's take a look at how the mother may respond unproductively or productively to the more cooperative e-mail that was sent. For the sake of developing this character, let's say that she was in a relationship with the child's father, and was left for another woman when she announced the pregnancy.

The unproductive response:

> *You lied to me. You cheated on me. You left me after I announced that our planned attempts for me to get pregnant were successful. As far as I'm concerned, a liar and a cheater is all you will ever be, and I don't want my child to be raised by a cheating liar. And no, of course you can't be at the hospital! And the paternity test: You know damned well that I am not the one who cheated! If you want a paternity test, you're going to have to fight for it. And the only way any of your whores will have any contact with or access to my child is over my dead body. Take a hike, loser.*

Do you see what is wrong here? Although we can understand her anger, and there is a part of us that wants to cheer for her determination and see her "win" this fight, the fact is, if this is how she plays, unless she is a multi-millionaire who can pick up and start anew in a different state and use her money to hire lawyers in a potentially unending legal battle, she will lose.

First of all, nothing in this e-mail is about the baby, but is instead all about her: the anger and resentment that she is—rather understandably—holding on to. She did not give the baby's father a clear understanding of what he would need to do in order to move forward, but instead told him clearly that he was shut out (and as we will see later in this chapter, a verbal warning will most often compromise the effectiveness of any shut-out strategy).

Bear in mind that giving the "appropriate response" (below) will also very likely flush out anyone who is truly not interested in working things out for the benefit of the child and an effective co-parenting relationship. If you can have the same results by holding yourself high than you can through being snarky, choose the option that will not hurt you in the long run.

The productive response:

> *Thank you for the letter. I recognize your intention to be a father and do intend to talk to you when I am ready, but for now I appreciate the opportunity to continue this pregnancy without any unnecessary contact. I am still processing the fact that you left me as soon as I became pregnant, and I need time to heal from that in order to deal with you without anger, as that wouldn't be good for any of us. Right now, the baby is in my body, and undue stress can damage us both, so I am protecting us both when I ask that you give us space. I will contact you when I am ready.*

Let's say our fictitious mother-to-be is ready to let the baby's father know the terms she expects in order to have smooth relations as co-parents.

> *Thank you for the letter. I recognize your intention to be a father. In order for things to be smooth between us, I am going to ask that you be fair in your financial investment and personal commitment to the baby. This will help even out our playing field, and will help close the door on some of the injustices that took place so that we can truly put an end to them and move forward.*

Do be advised that once paternity is established, I will seek child support, which in most cases is a standard twenty percent of your income, as well as half of my labor and delivery costs, and also—because I will have to work—an agreed-upon percentage of my child care costs on top of that (depending on available options and to be renegotiated when he/ she goes to kindergarten), while giving me the ultimate choice in where the baby goes for care. Additionally, since your job has better insurance than mine, I will request that the baby be added to your insurance policy upon receipt of the paternity test. All of this should be legally formalized, and your child support collected through the child support enforcement office. I will request your cooperation in getting this expedited quickly.

I am also requesting that you show up on time to any scheduled visitations, which will be supervised at least for the first year—that if you fail to show up, you agree to give me $25 for each portion of an hour that you are late (example: Ten minutes late= $25.00, one hour and ten minutes late= $50.00), payable immediately, or your future visitations are canceled—and that this is documented in writing.

I'm sure that through your research you are aware that agreeing peacefully to these terms will be far less costly than litigation.

I am also requesting that all of these conditions be met for the first five years of our child's life, at which time we may discuss whether you want or can handle having partial custody. Before that time, if we can work peacefully together, I will likely agree to your having extended time with our child—but first you have to demonstrate that you are responsible and consistent.

There will be other conditions that I will require in order for us to work together, but I first want to see what you think of the most important things—if we can't agree on this, it is doubtful that we can agree on anything else. But do know that I am willing to work things out in a way that benefits us all without compromising my autonomy or authority as a parent.

For your protection as well as mine, I request that we formalize our agreement in a legally-filed co-parenting agreement. This will help us to avoid any future litigation which can be expensive, and will help ensure that our initial agreements will not be forgotten and will be adhered to.

I hope you will see that this would be a start in the right direction so we can work well together in our child's life.

As you can see, this woman was firm, and required what was fair, but was not personally insulting. If this letter were read by a judge, this mother would seem knowledgeable, level-headed, and mature. The father would have a clear idea of what he needed to do in order for the situation to heal.

If sending a letter such as this one earns a retaliatory response, print it up and file it (or file it electronically), and respond with, "These are my terms, and they represent what is economically fair. They are not up for negotiation." Let him respond again and again if he likes, and respond the same way every time. Do not get dragged into debate. Keep it firm and non-personal, and keep all his correspondence.

In the event that he does come back into your life as a partner, which can happen when a man learns that you are not an easy nut to crack, stay the course, and keep finances separate. If that's not possible, keep documentation of your expenses versus his, and all the money he gives you for child support. That way, if his involvement in your life was just a ruse or was the most viable current option, you will not likely lose any ground, legally speaking.

If You Need Time to Heal Before Communication

If you are still chagrined about injustices that occurred within the relationship, take some time to process your wounds before agreeing to regular communication and cooperation.

If the father becomes impatient with your request to take this time, and his communication becomes threatening and abusive, then all bets are off. Some people can put on a good act for a certain amount of time and then lose it. Threatening communication needs to be ignored (bear in mind that actual physical threats, including threats to sabotage your job or find you in public, need to be put to rest through a restraining order). If it garners a response, you are training him to threaten you. Instead, train him to communicate with respect.

Protecting Yourself

Even if you are going through a time of smooth and effective communication, you must always protect yourself: As anyone who has been down this road will tell you, peaceful times don't always last. Sometimes the child's father will marry a woman who is threatened by the idea of peaceful co-parenting, and then he must choose between keeping you happy and keeping peace in his own home. Sometimes a person who was once functional will develop an addiction or some other harmful habit. Sometimes one parent or the other will have a work opportunity in another town, and then the war for physical custody is on. Sometimes a parent will agree to something they simply have no intention of following through with in order to get what they want in the moment. Sometimes people will simply change.

Following are a few rules of conduct—regardless of whether communication is smooth or contentious—to help you get and keep a good foothold on your situation.

Do not "Show your Cards."

You may be tempted to show a man your arsenal in order to demonstrate that it would be foolish to take you on, but all that does is let him know the arms he needs to amass in order to beat you. If you have spoken to an attorney, don't tell him! If your parents are bankrolling your attorney fees, don't tell him! If you have advocates who are advising you, don't tell him! If you know that he has been hanging out with criminals, don't tell him! If you have a list of tasks and responsibilities that identify you as the child's primary caregiver that you plan to share in the event that you go to court, don't share it with him! Only reveal what is required of you at the time that it becomes required.

Conversely, if he shows any of his cards to you, take note. If he says he has an attorney, then get a free consultation with every attorney in town, starting with the most ruthless. An attorney cannot work for him if they have prior knowledge of the case. If he claims that he should be the primary caregiver because he has ample financial resources, take note of that in the event that you seek child support. If he voices plans to move and take the child with him, be sure to work a "no move" clause into any interim agreement that is slated to lead towards joint custody. If he has family in another country that is not party to the Hague Convention and would like to take the child there, make sure to leave the father's name of the birth certificate, take steps towards obtaining the child's passport as soon as possible, and hire an expert to make a statement regarding child abductions to that country. If he is trying to intimidate you, silently thank him for the opportunity to give him rope. Let him reveal his plans while you keep yours a secret.

Unless a judge orders unsupervised visitation, don't hand him anything. Let him do his own research on issues like custody, visitation, caregiving, paternity testing, and child support enforcement. Educate yourself, but let him come to the table either educated or not—this will show how serious he truly is.

Do all that you can to work out your agreement without involving litigation, but do make sure any agreement is legally documented or filed with the appropriate agency so that they must be adhered to. Don't sacrifice your assets to fight a war when you can instead negotiate a very inexpensive peace treaty. Be strategic, be fearless, and learn to keep secrets. This is how you succeed.

The Single Woman's Guide to a Happy Pregnancy

Let Him Walk

If your baby's father refuses or fails to engage in discussion or communication, document the last time you spoke, and do not try to contact him or go after him insisting that he talk with you. Let him walk. Whether you ultimately want to work out a co-parenting situation or not, whether you plan to seek child support or not—or whatever your plans may be—you are giving up your control of the situation by chasing him. Let him write his own story—don't write it for him. You've got your own story to write a happy ending for.

Do Not Engage in Threats of Any Kind

You will become hyper-aware of what a threat is. In other words, "If you do/ don't do this, this will happen to you/ I will do this to you." Threats put a person on the defensive, which encourages counter-attacks. Instead, phrase your demands differently: "This is what needs to happen because this is what's fair." "This is what needs to happen in order to establish a peaceful working relationship between us." Furthermore, when you tell the baby's father what needs to happen, stand your ground. If you waver at all, he will see the cracks. This is one reason to take enough time to heal and get solid before you tell him what needs to be done.

Remember: This is not Personal—it's Business

What are the benefits of working out a peaceful co-parenting relationship with a responsible and non-dangerous man? Well, there's the child support. There's also the potential free babysitting and the extra free time you can have when you know your child is in good hands (bear in mind this is *only* a benefit if you are confident that your baby *is* in good hands, so your example of high conduct must be willingly met in order for this to be an advantage). There is also the potential bonus of better insurance from your child's father. Additionally, there are more relatives, more friends, and more people taking pride and investing in the child's accomplishments.

Learn to keep business and personal separate. If you had started a successful business and then wanted a partner to join you, would you let them jump on without making the appropriate financial investment? Of course not! If the business were to fail, you would be the only one to truly suffer. If a business partner has not shown good faith with the initial investment, you'd be a fool to let them in. But if they have, you don't have to completely approve of their every personal action in order to work with them—you just have to believe that they will do their best at the job, and that their best will be good enough.

This is another reason to do what you can to make sure your wounds are properly healed, and make sure the father is willing to do his part in that by enforcing that the negotiations of co-parenting are not a struggle. In order for this project to work, it has to be about working together.

Once those wounds are healed and the emotions are put to rest, conduct your communication as though it were one hundred percent business. If he misses a visitation, that is not something that should make you hurt or angry—it should instead be something that puts money in your pocket and teaches your child's father that there are consequences to being flaky that have nothing to do with how anyone "feels."

Set yourself up so that you can keep your "eyes on the prize" for your child instead of nursing old wounds. (Note: Never use the term "eyes on the prize" in court. Judges generally hate that.)

Never Mention your Struggles

If the man cannot see the struggles a woman will incur when she is left pregnant and alone, it's not likely that he will begin to understand them after she has pointed them out. The fact is most men in this country deny that patriarchy exists at all, and no amount of education is going to change that until a recognized injustice is suffered by one of his female loved ones. And no matter what things look like right now, when someone has contributed to injustice via patriarchy, karma will come around.

Trying to get your child's father to understand your feelings, your hurt, your sacrifice, or society's imbalance will get you two places: angry and nowhere. Thus, don't ask him for justice—instead, demand fairness as a condition of your participation. If you don't get it, don't play. If he wants to be in your child's life, he'll learn soon enough how that can be accomplished.

Cooperation and Trust are Two Different Things

Just because he is cooperating does not mean you can relax. One thing that you will hear said by mothers of toddlers and small children is this: It's too quiet in there—I have to check on them to make sure they're not doing anything naughty! Sometimes, just like toddlers, underdog parents will be "quiet" (peaceful) when something is in the works.

A real-life example: Jennie's son's father was being uncharacteristically cooperative when she found out that he had been embezzling her son's college fund. At the time the account was opened, her child's father had insisted that the bank statements go to his house because he (in his own words) "didn't trust her." To prove to him that embezzlement was a non-issue to her, she agreed. A year before finding out about the embezzlement, she had been notified that her son's bank had done away with the two-signature requirement (signatures of both parents) in order to withdraw from his savings account. Her son's father had put on such a show that they needed a two-signature account, implying that she was not to be trusted. Assuming that he would autonomously want to prove his own trustworthiness in this situation, and road-weary from too many conflicts, she neglected to facilitate the moving of her son's money. Two years later, after very few confrontations and generally smooth interactions, she found that her son's account had been all but drained.

When she confronted her son's father, his response was, "Why do you have to get all mad? It will be returned. You *know* that." She knew no such thing. When she pressed the issue, the nastiness returned. They had to go to court. There was peace again until one day she checked to find that he was two months late on his payments.

Thankfully, the courts agreed that the account needed to be reconstituted. But every time Jennie made her son's father aware of her knowledge that he was late on a payment, the personal game would commence again: "You are bitter." "Can't you see I'm poor?" "If you insist on causing problems…" or he would say something vague, like "dealt with," which to her implied that a deposit had been made. Days later, she'd check. No deposit had been made.

Like Jennie's son's father, many men will dangle the idea of peace over your head under the condition that you turn a blind eye to what is wrong. This is not cooperating, it' manipulating. Always watch your back. Set a standard, and stick to it. And do not be emotionally manipulated. Remember: This is business.

Resist Temptation to Insult the Other Party, Even if it's Subtle
You may think you are being clever when you slip a well-hidden slight in your e-mail communication, but all this will serve to do is hurt you. After all, your child's father may not be very smart, but let's hope that any judge who ends up reading these e-mails *is* smart (and decent). Although we have all been tempted and many have acted upon it, to slight your child's father is clearly inciting conflict and wanting to "win" rather than working towards a solution. If he subscribes to this type of communication, he is shooting himself in the foot, and I advise that communication be cut off. Don't ever make yourself the villain.

Beware the Ruse
Many times when a person makes an issue of something, it is an attempt to ensure that nobody suspects them of what they are accusing the other party of.

Take for example the banking incident above. The mother was "not to be trusted." As a result she aimed to prove her trustworthiness rather than seeing the ruse, while the other party was embezzling the child's money.

In the case of another one of my counselees, someone (whom she suspects is her baby's father) reported her to child protective services as a drug abuser. She was required to immediately take a drug test under observation, which she passed, but it was a humiliating situation for her and confusing for her older children, who were interviewed about their mother's behavior. The suspicious component of the accusation is that the baby's father—who happened to be a surgeon who was bitter about paying more than two million dollars in child support over eighteen years—was a prescription drug abuser himself. When this counselee requested through the court that the baby's father take a hair follicle drug test (which will show a person's drug activity for the past three months) in order to have unsupervised visitation, he shaved his head. Is there any mystery as to why? Not to me. But possibly because the mother had engaged in too much debate, and had even temporarily gotten back together with the father while knowing of his habits (or unfortunately, possibly because the judge simply did not like women), her accusation was regarded as retaliation against his rejection rather than legitimate concern for her child's well-being. He was awarded 50 percent custody, which he didn't even want.

That said, pay very close attention to those "accusations." Your response (when it's possible), "I will if he will." Also, make sure that when you accuse someone else of a certain behavior, that you are not guilty of that same behavior yourself. Again, "I will if he will." Additionally, if someone's behavior is potentially dangerous (as in drug abuse), you need to be the first one to act on it. Your motives will be under question if you do not.

Turn the Page

If you have made any of the abovementioned mistakes up to this point, don't panic. Simply redefine yourself. Write one final correspondence to your child's father and send it (unless he has asked you not to contact him or has said he doesn't want to be involved, in which case you write it and keep it until he contacts you) using the guidelines I have outlined in this chapter.

If he does contact you, send the letter—unless he is combative and insulting. If he is, you have two choices: leave him in the dust, or send a non-combative response that sets the tone for the communication you expect, and see if that works. If he responds with anger or insults, file that correspondence, and stop contacting him.

Being Careful about Social Media

Social media is important to lots of people, especially those who are somewhat socially shut in due to a pregnancy or a new baby. However, what you say or do on social media can compromise you in a lot of ways. Although it's tempting to use social media as your personal venting platform, you must resist disseminating personal information to a wide audience—some of whom may also be friends with your adversaries. Even those people with the best of intentions can unknowingly say something that can ultimately hurt you.

I learned about the dangers of social media the hard way, and learned it twice: My first incident involved what some would call a suitor with very bad judgment, and others would call a stalker. A friend had brought my attention to the fact that someone had written a "missed connections" post about me on Craigslist (in case you don't know, this is where people post about having seen people in public—basically in hopes of meeting). I wondered how she could tell: There are hundreds of brown-haired women who drive a Saturn Vue and own a husky—how would anyone be able to tell a missed connections post was about *me*? When I looked on craigslist, I saw the post: My first name, last name, and location were the title of the post. Not flattering. I felt like my personal information just been written on the bathroom wall.

The post went on to say things like "I fantasize about staying up late and arguing over your anarcho-feministic philosophies." That bugged me. First of all, I don't stay up late unless I'm having fun, and I don't enjoy arguing; secondly, my opinions are perfectly reasonable, thank you, and they are not up for negotiation with some dude. Finally, the suitor refused to reveal his identity, other than that he was watching me on Facebook.

Yup, I was creeped out. So was the Internet Crimes unit at my local police department, and I've seen police ignore some pretty significant things. I was urged to report the incident and take some steps to ensure my privacy.

I had really enjoyed being a popular "microblogger." Everything I said got 100 likes within minutes, and I had some great, productive discussions—it really inflated the heck out of my ego. I tried to salvage my friends list by deleting and blocking a few people, somewhat concerned that I might be deleting an elderly relative, an old college friend's kid, or the supportive boyfriend or father of one of my readers. I found that I could not change or delete past work history, places lived, or contact information. I ultimately scrapped my page, created another one under a fictitious name using an underused email address as the only contact information, used a photo of my dog as my profile picture (everyone who knew me knew my dog), and re-invited who I thought were my real friends. Interestingly, when I did this, someone reported me as someone who they didn't know, and Facebook threatened to shut my page down.

The worst part of this is that some porn sites take Craigslist Missed Connections posts and re-post them on their sites in order to get traffic—so when I was googling myself to make sure the post had been deleted, I found my first name, last name, and location right next to an amateur photo of a woman showing her genitals and headlines of "hot singles want to meet you in your town," or something like that. I was able to get the sites to take the post down, but it was a bit scary in the interim.

The second incident involved my single pregnancy Facebook page—but while it is a painful memory, this story can also show how easy it is to find information about someone. While working at a magazine, I was complaining about all the company executives who beg me to write about them while supporting anti-mother initiatives. Well, somebody saw that: A "company executive who wished to remain anonymous" swiftly wrote a several-page letter to my boss calling for a stiff reprimand, if not termination.

Interestingly, as I later found, it was NOT a company executive, but rather a former friend who had strong opinions about my work and mission. We'd had a falling out that, in my experience, was not so dramatic. I simply stopped contacting her. I had no idea she had been stewing.

As my immediate supervisor was rather naïve about human resources matters, the name of the complainer was revealed to me. The writer pretended she was a man named Mac Welch. Believing that a man had been watching me was pretty disturbing after my Facebook stalking fiasco. I searched the Internet for someone named Mac Welch—it became apparent that this was a pseudonym.

About a week later, I noticed that I had a twitter follower named Mac Welch. The profile was blank, but "Mac" was following one other person, apparently a young adult who seemed to party pretty hard. I looked this other person up on Facebook and found his location: Same home town as the abovementioned former friend, and some of his Facebook friends shared her unusual maiden name. I looked up how many people shared that name in the United States: very few. I remembered how she spied on the young people in her extended family to make sure they weren't getting into too much trouble. Then I got the code: "Mac," the first letters of her current last name, "Welch," the last name of her favorite singer.

I briefly contacted her, and let her know the jig is up. Then I blocked her from all my social media. I learned my lesson too: Just because someone is a "fan" of your page, doesn't mean that they like you or are on your side. Everything you say on social media should be something that cannot in any way come back to hurt you. You may be surprised at who is watching and waiting for that opportunity.

You might ask yourself, as I have, who the heck would do all of this? The answer: Weirdos! And yes, they are out there in spades. Don't they have anything better to do? For some people, internet voyeurism is a very satisfying compulsion. It is extremely important to make sure that none of your sensitive information can leak to the wrong people on Facebook or other social media sites.

At the time of this writing, Facebook and Twitter are the dominant social media, although my son insists that Facebook is for "old people," and that Instagram, Snapchat, Tumblr, and Kik are "what everybody is doing" these days (it should be noted that he refers to Kik as "nude photo central." Note: Because such things can always be used against her to destroy her career and social standing, a woman should never, ever share nude photos with anyone unless she is a professional model under contract. Any man worthy of seeing you nude will respect that boundary, or he needs to be let go.) Since I am in no way an expert on most social media, I will focus on practices that you can apply to social media in general, in hopes that you will be able to apply the same standards to the media you use.

Anonymity, using various Social Media as examples
Facebook

Facebook is always changing. If you cannot delete or block people without bringing attention to yourself, start a new account and use a fake name and profile/cover images that only your friends will recognize. Write to those friends personally and tell them who you are if you don't think they will get it. You can have Facebook download the entirety of your old content for you before you shut it down, and (at the time of this writing) your old profile will be there if you ever log back in under your old log-in, so nothing is lost.

Do not give any more information than is required—at the time of this writing, that's an e-mail address. Do not reveal where you work, where you live, or your phone number (no matter how many times it is asked for and why). Where you went to school: your choice. Put the security settings on high, and at this point you can even hide things that you don't want certain friends to see. Make sure you have the ability to approve any photo or post in which you are tagged, and make sure people can't post on your timeline. Block anyone you don't trust from seeing your new profile. Only invite people who are *your* friends (not shared between you and your baby's father), and still, only say decidedly positive or neutral things. Try not to generalize about or bash the opposite gender in the posts or memes you share, because this may alienate true friends and attract men that do the same to women. Any venting is to be done privately with trusted friends and family, or anonymously through an online group—not publicly on your Facebook page. If you are not certain of a friend's integrity, manage your profile so that they can't see everything. If people are sure to say things that upset you, you can keep them as a friend, but hide their posts.

Turn off the location feature on your smartphone, and never say publicly where you are. This can prevent you from being sabotaged or tracked down in public. Also, there are apps that essentially help predators get personal information about women from their social media pages while disclosing their locations. This way, they can ask about your brother and your dog, and give you the idea that they know you, sometimes to make a more-or-less innocent although dishonest connection—but sometimes not. This is scary, but it won't happen if your locator is turned off, if you use a fake name on your profile, and if your profile photo is a picture of your pet bird and your cover photo is scenery. If you do all three, someone might still be able to locate you, but not likely through a social media app.

LinkedIn

LinkedIn is one social media app that is meant to enhance professional connections rather than social ones. It does not make sense to have a LinkedIn profile that does not feature a complete history of where you have worked, and it is also ideal that you have your most professional portrait on your profile.

Use your discretion with LinkedIn. People cannot see your history if you are not a connection, but they will be able to see where you currently work.

On LinkedIn, I only accept connection requests from individuals—not businesses or people who do not provide their portrait and seem legitimate enough through having a logical collection of connections and a disclosed work history.

While LinkedIn is popular in the business community, I have yet to see its benefit other than to show which important person you have done business with—or not (many people send contact requests despite never having met or worked with you), although some people claim that it can be used to recruit employees or find a job. If showing your portrait and disclosing your place of work is risky, just don't do it. I personally feel that to have fewer social media accounts, all of which are truly useful to you, is much safer than having several accounts.

Cafemom.com

As the owner of a group on Cafemom.com, I know it can be extremely helpful to find a diverse group of compassionate, supportive, and knowledgeable women who can give grounded advice and want to see you succeed. I also know that it can be extremely damaging to bear your heart to strangers and be judged, or to read endless posts that condemn people of your race, political views, spiritual views, income level, or marital status—which is something I have witnessed in some of the public groups. The first bit of advice I have about Cafemom.com is to find groups that reflect your specific interests, and stay away from groups where people are judging, fighting, and being unproductive. Being reminded that such people exist can certainly deflate your attitude for a day—or more. People can post anonymously, so they can dodge accountability for their harmful words, sit back, and watch the show. Some people enjoy being destructive and judgmental. Although it would be unsafe to forget that such people exist, avoid them at all costs. Your energy needs to be focused on the good in this world.

My second bit of advice is about your personal privacy and security. Just like with any online group or social media, it is a good idea not to post a photo of yourself or have any personal clues in your screen name. Although I, as a group owner, usually screen group applicants to make sure they are actually single pregnant women and not women seeking children to adopt (some of whom have pretended to be single pregnant women when they had applied to be in the support group), I did accidentally let a baby daddy into the group one time. He had made a profile complete with photographs. Thankfully, this was not a dangerously volatile situation—but as you can imagine, nor was it ideal. I could not have investigated the applicant more thoroughly without potentially invading the privacy of a woman who might already have been traumatized by having to defend herself against CPC counselors, family, or her child's father.

So remember that just because someone has your back, that does not necessarily mean they know what they are doing. Always use fake names for yourself and your children until you have developed a personal relationship with someone. If you discuss your location, do so anonymously: "I'm from a small town in Michigan." Your first line of defense is always yourself. Everyone else is back-up.

Shutting the Father out
The decision to shut the father out is as personal as the decision to have a baby in the first place. There are many reasons why someone might take this course, and there is no "one-size-fits-all" set of circumstances that necessitates taking this action. Although shutting the father out is often harshly judged in the court of public opinion, I have only seen this option used (or more accurately, attempted) in a handful of cases where I didn't feel it was the best option for the mother and child—and let's face it: If a man wants to be a father, he needs to be cooperative, mature, and take initiative. If he is nowhere to be found, he probably wants it that way. We know the advantages of having a co-parent to a child. If those advantages don't seem worth the trouble, they probably aren't. Some people will say things like, "Sure, he disappears and loses contact for long periods of time, but does that mean he shouldn't be a father?" My answer: Fathers are present for and accessible to their kids. You can't just walk away and leave your child at home for a few hours… a day… a week—the child would die. Even houseplants need more than this in order to survive. Why should the father be able to do such a thing? Or, "He is late or altogether misses his visitations, but does that mean he should lose his rights?" Well, an employee can lose their job—their livelihood—for the same. If a mother is depending on his punctuality for her survival, the answer to that is, yes. And finally, as we have mentioned before, it is not the mother's job to raise a man—it is her job to raise the child. If the father gets in the way of her economic and parenting success, he is no asset. If she is even capable of shutting him out without having to relocate to a different town, he is not present or committed enough to be an asset.

I maintain that women who use this option are, for the most part, doing so justly. Occasionally I meet someone who wants to use the shut-option for vengeance or attention, but if that's the case, they usually falter in their resolve.

In order for the shut-out to work, the mother has to want it with every fiber of her being. It is not a game or a joke. A woman can't go half-way down the shut-out road and then turn around—to do so rips open wounds, weakens boundaries, drags out the drama, and can sometimes create a dangerous situation. She must be one hundred percent ready to close the book and start another. Her decision has to be about her safety, economic health, and personal freedom, and/or that of the child.

If it is going to work, it cannot be an act of vengeance. It cannot be to teach a person a lesson. When we engage in vengeance towards another person, it spiritually and energetically links us to them, and then they have a way of sticking to our shoes. A person's actions will always catch up with them. The goal is not to ensure that another person suffers for what they have done, but rather to be too busy doing something productive with your own life to notice when their actions catch up with them. As many say, "God has a plan." If you subscribe to this belief, have faith that God has a plan for him as well as for you. His will come with its own set of challenges and regrets.

Some have done it to show the world that they were "not in it for the money" in cases where the child's father is rich. Again, the shut-out is not about proving anything to anyone else. If a woman is shutting a man out to "prove" anything to herself or anyone else, I have to assert that this is a bad reason. If someone thinks you are doing something for the money, it's normally because they themselves would do it for the money—and frankly, they are jealous that you might get some. But if the man is angry, bitter, or resistant, a man with lots of money can also be a formidable adversary, so this situation would need to be handled with care.

Additionally, it cannot be a cry for attention. If it is, it might work and it might not, but it will certainly set the stage for drama either way. You also cannot give an ultimatum. If you say things like, "this is your last chance to be a father or I am going to disappear," it is obvious that you have given him enough chances already, and he is simply not interested—to beat against that door is to play a childish game. Yes, he might be making a big mistake, but let his mistakes be his own—not yours. If you make threats to control the situation rather than simply controlling it, you are going to engage him in a war and have a lot more attention than you ever wanted—all of it negative.

Thus, the shut out is not to be taken lightly. The decision must be firm. All doors must be sealed and locked.

In some situations, the shut out can be simple and easy: Don't contact him.

In others, it takes a bit more effort: Change your phone number and your email, delete (and re-start, if you like) your social media, and don't contact him.

More dangerous situations require more drastic action: Change residences, change phone number and email, delete social media, and don't contact him. If that won't do the trick, follow all the same steps, and leave town. You may even consider leaving the state or leaving the country, if you have an appropriate situation to go to.

If you have a protective order against the father, follow all these steps, and make a plan to move as soon as it expires—this way, the authorities will not have to report to him where you are (in order to observe the protective order), and you will not have left a trail for him to follow.

At this point, I hope I don't have to reiterate that you should leave his name off the birth certificate. I am of the school of thought that the birth certificate should never be mentioned to the child's father regardless of your plans because it can compromise your freedom in many ways. If the father does not initiate the birth certificate discussion, the option to sign should never be handed to him. As with everything, if the father wants to be on the birth certificate, he will seek that honor—his name can always be added later, and is sometimes added by court order (at the father's expense) after a child support and custody settlement has been reached. In my opinion, it should never be added without these two things in place.

If the Gum Sticks to your Shoes
Sometimes, no matter how hard you try, no matter how many rules you follow, you still end up in court litigating a parenting arrangement with a contentious opposing party.

This is where all of your past actions and behaviors can come back to serve you well, or bite you in the ass. Do not be scared, but do not be overly confident either. If it has gotten to this place, it's anybody's game—but always play the best you can on your first go-round because it's much easier to establish something that serves you from the start than it is to modify or undo something that has been established.

Dealing with Attorneys
I'll be honest with you: A good attorney is hard to find. I had two bad attorneys before my childhood friend returned to our home town and showed me what my last two had done so wrong. Most attorneys will let you believe that their services are more necessary than they are, and will drag out any court proceedings in order to line their pockets while you end up with an agreement that is dissatisfactory. It is important to do as much research as you can before hiring an attorney—and while it is wise to follow a trusted attorney's advice, remember that they work for *you*.

Attorneys will always require a retainer, which is a certain amount of money, maybe two or three thousand dollars or what you will ultimately owe her, paid up-front to make sure the initial work she does is not for nothing (at least not for *her*). If you think there is any possibility of having to go to court, this is a good reason to start saving *now*.

Following are some recommendations for finding a drama-free attorney and helping make sure things happen right for you.

1. Many family law attorneys provide free initial consultations. Seek as many free consultations as you can before deciding on an attorney. An attorney can't represent your child's father if he or she has prior knowledge of the case, so seeking as many consultations before you hire an attorney can help you in many ways. Always

consult with the attorneys with the nastiest reputations first, so your baby's father can't ultimately hire them. Always pretend you haven't spoken to anyone else and listen closely to what their plan of action would be with your case.
2. During the consultation, ask the attorney how much experience he or she has with custody and child support agreements between parents where the mother and father were never married. Your situation can be very different from custody and child support as the result of divorce.
3. Ask if there are things that can be done by you personally—papers filed with the court, for example—in order to save money. There's no reason to pay $300 for your attorney to have her paralegal do something that you can do yourself. Ask that you attorney tell you when there are opportunities to cut costs.
4. Ask what he or she thinks are the most important aspects of your dissatisfaction with your child's father (he has been verbally violent and threatening, he is a known drug dealer, etc.). See if your attorney can pinpoint what will and will not be taken seriously by the judge.
5. Ask the attorney whether you think the judge assigned to your case will be sympathetic or if they have a record of patriarchal decisions.
6. Mediation can often be less costly than court, but should only be attempted if you have peace with your child's father—and if attorneys are involved, my opinion is that there isn't enough peace for a fair mediation. Still, if you are prepared and do not budge with what is important to you, this may work out.
7. If you file a motion (a request that a judge issue a ruling on a legal matter) for custody, for example, and your baby's father files an opposition (response) that brings up a series of irrelevant details about the situation, this is an attempt to distract you from your goal, drain your energy, and diminish your finances. Request that your case go straight to court rather than allowing this to be a long-term expensive mess.
8. If your child's father files a motion against you, request that your attorney deem his motion a frivolous law suit meant to further diminish the resources you and your child need to live as a retaliatory measure, and request that your attorney fees and half your pregnancy medical bills be paid by your child's father in addition to any support. Furthermore, request that the case go to court as soon as possible. In other words, if he fires the first shot, burn the bridge and bomb the village.

Make no mistake about it: Court is frightening. Do not be overly confident that you will get your desired outcome, no matter how good you are and how much support you've received from family, friends, your community, or the community. You may have heard that courts often side with the mother and that fathers most often get the raw deal. Well, here's the very bad news: This is more true in the event that the parents were married. Married women followed society's rules by not having children until married, and the father in this situation is often viewed as someone who did not hold up his end of the marriage deal. With a single pregnant woman, there was never any official legal deal that the father abandoned. This is one reason why you need to do your very best to show that you are a responsible honest, stable person from the moment you begin this process to the end.

Bear in mind that judges are individuals. Some have a history of being compassionate towards single mothers, and some feel that we are a burden upon society. Some feel they are always doing something positive by encouraging co-parenting, even if the two parties involved can't communicate civilly to save their lives. If you have an attorney, ask the attorney what kind of experience they have with that judge and what the judge's history is. You can often request to change the judge on your case one time, but can sometimes get a worse judge than the one you had.

If you happen to end up in court and made some mistakes in your conduct before you read this book, you can often defend yourself from your past actions by using a point of reference in time: "Once I realized that I am going to have a child and need to care for that child, I changed my behavior," or, "I was extremely traumatized/wounded/frightened by the events immediately leading up to that point, but I have since re-stabilized and understand the importance of facing these challenges calmly." If the father is able to pay child support but is dysfunctional in another crucial way, and still insists on being a part of the child's life, he should likewise be kept away from the child if possible. However, although there are exceptions, the courts will generally not enforce that the father stay away for many reasons that a mother may find dangerous or damaging.

In court, do your best not to focus on annoyances and minor injustices. If you focus on these things, you will be regarded as a troublemaker, and the quickest way to get them to stop is to stop giving them energy through paying attention to them. I know of a very sad case where the mother was granted sole physical custody and had to let the father have unsupervised visitation two days a week. This caused her extreme anxiety—she was a very conscientious mother, and the father was an unsavory character, although he was not obviously breaking any laws. She was extremely uncooperative. One time she refused to hand her child over for his unsupervised visitation for no specific reason, just that he had an evil look in his eye. When she went back to court, she mentioned the fact that her child was afraid of his father, and expressed anger that he had repeatedly failed to return the child's security blanket, which honestly may very well have been to antagonize her. However, exhausted by the drama, the judge granted the father partial custody, and told her that if she refused to hand the child over one more time, no matter the reason, he would get sole custody. The mother's legitimate concerns were eclipsed by blanket drama, and she suffered dearly.

Sometimes a judge will assign a visitation arrangement knowing full well that the father will fail to follow the order. In cases such as this, do not express disappointment. Simply document the failures. When you revisit the court case, be sure not to exhibit anger and emotion. Just the facts, ma'am: The court order was not followed.

Following is a list of things that I have come across that have normally been taken seriously, and those that have not.

Traits that may be considered damaging enough to deny custody:

> *Criminal activity*
> *Unresolved addiction* (including porn addiction, gambling addiction)
> *Illegal activity*
> *Lack of knowledge* (of how to care for an infant, for example)
> *Inability to communicate peacefully/co-parent* (save those e-mails and keep your own nose clean!)
> *Living with/regular contact with criminals*
> *Unsanitary living conditions*
> *Missing scheduled meetings*, especially causing the mother to miss work
> *Bad credit*
> *Domestic violence history*
> *Involvement in groups that practice sado-masochism or body mutilation,* especially those in which the participants don't use their real names or are otherwise anonymous (this is only taken seriously if you were never a participant)
> *Abandonment* (Bear in mind that abandonment means different things to different people, but sometimes a one-year absence from any contact is considered abandonment. Every state varies in its definition—do some research to find out the definition in your state. Also bear in mind that it's not abandonment if you tell him to leave. Thus, when he walks, always let him walk. Never chase him.)
> *Polyamory* (Remember that if you accepted it at one time in your relationship, it is often considered a non-issue.)

Some things that are brought up in court will not stand up on their own. If you refuse to work cooperatively with a child's father for the following reasons—while he remains determined to be involved in the child's life—you may be the one who comes out of the situation seeming like the one who is refusing to cooperate. Note: I am not saying that this is right *or* wrong, I'm just saying that it's the way it normally is.

Traits that will generally not be taken seriously on their own (but may bolster other issues):

> *Infidelity/ Polyamory* (if never accepted throughout your relationship)
> *A difference in religion or spiritual practices*
> *A difference in culture/heritage*
> *A failure to adhere to high nutrition/ medical care standards*
> *Lack of steady employment* (although a father with no money can often not afford to take the issue of custody to court, so this can sometimes be a wash)
> *A difference in parenting philosophies* (these should be addressed and agreed upon in a co-parenting agreement rather than assumed to be a reason not to co-parent)
> *Father's family involved in criminal activity*
> *Father is in a relationship with the woman he left you for/a new woman* and is touting her importance as a female role model or their importance as a functioning two-parent family

No matter the situation, you can usually come out of a court conflict with a satisfying agreement if you maintain control over your emotions and keep your cool.

◆ ◆ ◆

As you can see, the lesson in this chapter is to hold yourself high for your child as well as yourself. In order to be an effective parent, you need to minimize unnecessary distractions or challenges and maximize your resources. In order to have a good future, you need to focus on what is productive and supportive. Remember: When you are a parent, you are both a sentry and an example, but not everybody sees those roles in the same way, and every situation is unique. Take enough time to yourself to make the right decision and take the best action for your future and that of your child.

Chapter Eight

Do I Really Need a Bassinet?

Frankly, there are things that you will *need*, and there are things that you will *want*, but are the things you will want really the things you will *use*? Aha! Food for thought! When you truly know what you do and don't need as well as what will truly help, you can minimize waste and increase efficiency. In this chapter, I will first discuss the pros and cons of certain popular baby items, and then I'll give you (most likely) your first truly honest bare-bones list of what you will need right away.

Things You May Never Need (But read the descriptions so you know why)
Believe it or not, you may never need a crib! Although those mysterious people "in the know" change their minds every so often about whether or not it's safe for your baby to sleep in your bed with you, I found that my son's crib was just a major waste of my space and it ended up permanently residing at my mother's house.

The speculations regarding the safety of your child sleeping in your bed are as follows: A few years ago, it was concluded that children are less likely to fall victim to Sudden Infant Death Syndrome (SIDS) if they sleep with their mothers because listening to someone else breathing is said to help them regulate their own breathing. At the time it was also said that women only seem to end up rolling on their babies and killing them if they are incredibly drunk. However, recently I heard on a TV morning news program that SIDS is more likely to occur if a child sleeps in bed with his parents, due to their blankets cutting off its air supply. Due to all this confusing information (although I am no scientist), I am going to go out on a limb and express my opinion on this matter: Sleeping with your child and SIDS are totally unrelated! Every family within my circle of friends (that includes two-parent families as well as one-parent families) has come upon circumstances involving money, travel, space, medical issues, or parenting philosophies, that required that the child sleep in his parents' or mother's bed for an extended period of time. Not one of these children was ever squished by his parents, and none of them died of SIDS. And according to many natural parenting experts, babies are happier and feel more secure when they're very close to their mothers.

Of course one must take measures to assure the child's safety while sleeping in your bed (see list on the bare bones of what you'll need right away), but I've been told that breastfeeding mothers whose babies sleep in their beds with them get a lot more sleep than those who do not breast feed. In addition, I feel that a good playpen is absolutely necessary for many reasons, and can be used as a crib on those occasions that you just need your bed to yourself.

Bassinets and cradles offer lovely ways to display your baby, but are outgrown so quickly that they might not be worth it, and although babies should be put in the reclining position for sleeping, too much time on the back is not recommended. Furthermore, does your home have room for all these different places for baby to sleep? Bassinets are nice because you can wheel them around and have the baby at your side no matter what you're doing, but I have found that a seat of some kind is a better choice because the baby can watch you while you tend to your taΩsks, which might also keep your baby entertained if he's of a certain temperament.

Humidifiers are only useful if you live in a dry climate, and even still, may never be necessary (I live in Alaska, which is very dry, and never needed one). In addition, they get filthy and have to be cleaned often. If you, your parents, or your pediatrician thinks your baby will benefit from humidity and you are not ready or able to buy, try heating some water in an electric kettle and pour the hot water in a pot, or boil a pot of water on the stove (but of course don't forget it's there) and throw some aromatic tea in it to make the house smell nice.

Swings, Jumpers, and Walkers: These are also hard novelties to judge. Some babies love them, and some hate them. It will all depend on your baby's preference. If you have friends who own these items, try them out before you consider buying them (if I had done this, I would have saved lots of money on that very nice swing my son hated). Always be cautious while using any of these items—just because the baby is happy and having fun doesn't mean that you don't have to pay attention. There have been numerous injuries and deaths of infants involving the improper or negligent use of walkers and jumpers. Despite their widespread use with newborn babies, swings are not recommended until the baby can hold his head up.

Changing Tables: Changing tables are very nice, especially for storage, but they are truly luxuries. Babies can be changed on a waterproof pad on the floor. If you have rowdy pets or otherwise feel that your floor is somehow unsafe, you can change the baby on your bed.

Disposable Diapers: Okay, I'll admit it: I have diaper issues. I'm a raging advocate of saving the environment, but I'm an even bigger advocate for saving the sanity of my fellow single mothers. Even for the most environmentally-conscious mothers, the answer lies in a careful blend of environmental sensitivity and facing the reality of your circumstances. The plain truth is this: There are certain times that disposable diapers make your life far easier, and every mother should have some disposables in her home even if she doesn't plan on using them regularly. It is a good idea to bring a couple of disposable diapers with you if you will be away from home for any extended period of time, whether your trip involves shopping, vacationing, staying at a friend's house, etc. As you will learn, sometimes you will change your baby after he's pooped, and then realize that he's not done, will change him again, and then realize that he still wasn't done!!! If you are away from home, always have more diapers than you think you will need.

You will also be required to provide disposable diapers if your child goes to day care. Biodegradable diapers are best, but can be expensive. Be easy on yourself, and understand that you have less time to do the things you need to do than a woman who has a partner. Even if you are a total Earth Mother, think of it as an environmental triumph every time you use a cloth diaper rather than a failure every time you use a disposable one.

Another limiting truth is this: cloth diapers will be much easier to manage if you have laundry facilities inside your home or within your building, or if your town has a diaper laundering service. If you have to take your clothes to a Laundromat, dragging a heavy load of soaked diapers down the block, on your day off, with your child in tow, is going to be hellish. Misery is the last thing you want right now.

However, for those of you determined to triumph, cloth diapers are much cheaper in the long run, they come in several different styles these days (most with Velcro closures and disposable pads for the inside, some of them even biodegradable), and are manageable with the right preparation. Depending on the brand and style you choose, they may have special laundering instructions (always save 800 numbers and informational contacts in case you have questions). However, following are basic instructions that provide safe laundering for **most** diaper styles (ask an authority before using Borax: it might not be considered safe to use on the particular brand of diapers you are using). All you need is a diaper pail (which will also be useful for soaking soiled garments), a toilet clean enough that you're not afraid to put your hands in it, and an inexpensive magical laundry additive known as Borax.

Note: some people assume that Borax is bleach because it is used to whiten laundry. It is NOT bleach; however, Borax should be used sparingly if your home has a septic system.

1. Rinse soiled diaper in the toilet, removing any solid residue.
2. Place diaper in a pail (with a secure lid) filled with 2 gallons of water and half cup of Borax, and allow them to soak until laundry time. Change diaper pail water and Borax (every one to three loads of laundry) at your discretion.
3. Machine wash.

Diaper Disposal System: You will only need a large plastic diaper pail if you're using cloth, but even if you're planning on exclusively using disposable diapers, *don't believe the hype*! You do not need an expensive diaper disposal system with the exclusive plastic refills that turn your baby's messy pants into big, white sausage links. These contraptions are wasteful for too many reasons to tell them all here. If a disposable diaper is merely pee-soaked, simply roll it up in a ball and attach the tape or Velcro so that it will not reopen. An effective and practical way to dispose of poopy diapers is to collect plastic bags from the supermarket and keep them in a box near where you change the baby (but out of his reach, of course), wrap the diaper in the plastic bag, knot it, and throw it away. Take out the trash regularly, and you should have no problem with bad smells.

Diaper Bags often come with pockets specifically designed for certain baby items, but I found backpack with several pockets will work just as well, will leave your arms and hands free, will still be useful years down the line, and most everyone has one lying around their house, or can acquire one cheaply.

Bibs: It is much more practical to get a couple of plastic bibs than to get several terry-cloth bibs. Plastic bibs can be rinsed or wiped clean and will not retain stains or require laundering. You can take them anywhere and they still do the trick. The best plastic bibs are the ones with snaps on the back rather than ties.

Infant Carriers: Both soft infant carriers and backpack-style carriers are useful in certain situations, but are completely useless in others. Slings are wonderful for newborns, but if your baby gains weight quickly (like mine did), it will not be appropriate for long-term use. Of course, this is not something you can anticipate. You may have to start using a more complex carrier quickly.

If you choose to use a more complex infant carrier in public, it is wise to have someone with you to help you, because for some people (especially those with a bad back or trick knees) it is virtually impossible to use the restroom while the baby is strapped in, and of course you can't leave the baby on the floor or on the public diaper deck. In addition, when you take the baby out of the carrier and are in a hurry to get him or her back into it, you may find yourself in a very frustrating situation if you can't figure out where the straps go and what attaches to what (always be very familiar with your equipment). Do lots of research and ask questions about soft infant carriers before you buy one or put one on your shower registry. Make sure you practice *a lot* with your infant carrier around the house before you go out with it, and make sure you know its limitations. Soft infant carriers are effective if you will just be running errands within walking distance of your home and need both hands free, if you need to do things around the house and don't want to put the baby down, if you're taking a walk near your house, or if you'll be taking public transportation from your house to a friend or relative's house; but they are not the best for all-day outings. In this case, you'll be better off using a stroller.

Shoes: Baby shoes are cute and are great for dress-up, but are really not recommended until the baby starts walking. However, many people think that the absence of shoes on a child (even if the child is not yet walking) is a comment on the negligent and lazy nature of the mother, and the last thing you need is some crazy person confronting you about your parenting abilities. This happened to me several times and trust me, it ruins your day, even if you know this person is full of it. It might be wise to invest in a couple of cloth shoes (with cloth soles) with laces, Velcro, or snaps to keep your child's feet covered.

Towels and Washcloths: Special towels and washcloths for your baby are cute, but are not necessary. Your own clean, soft towels and washcloths will do just fine.

Does it all have to match? No, there has never been any baby opinion poll concluding that babies are happiest looking at the same three colors all day. You may want to make your baby's environment as interesting as possible, but it does not have to subscribe to any canned color scheme.

Bottle Warmers are nice, but a cold bottle can simply be warmed by sitting it in hot water until it feels neither warm nor cold when you test the stream of the nipple against your wrist. You can also use slightly warm water when you're mixing formula. Some people use a microwave. I'm not a big fan of microwaves (don't even own one) because there is ongoing debate about whether it destroys nutrients, so I err on the side of caution. You can safely heat water in an electric kettle.

Mittens are probably the worst investment for your baby because they're always falling off. If you live in a cold climate, get suits that cover the baby's hands, feet, and head.

The Bare Bones of What You'll Need Right Away

It is wise to be ready for your baby before his due date, just in case your little one comes early. Throughout your pregnancy you will see several lists of what you'll need for your baby, and they will vary widely. Many of these lists don't take into account those women who are getting prepared with only one income, and many of them don't take into consideration that the amount of space available can be an issue, especially for single moms who either own or live in a rent-controlled studio or one- bedroom apartments in high-density urban settings like San Francisco or NYC.

You *will* want (and will end up with) much more than I've detailed in this list, but this is only meant to demonstrate the *minimum* of what you will need. In the pages to follow, I describe in detail what each item is and the important functions it performs.

A Place for the Baby to Sleep: This can be a crib, playpen, or even a spot next to you in your own bed. If you do put the baby in bed with you, make sure that:

> Your bed is large enough (at least a double)
> If your bed frame or mattress is against a wall, make sure your bed frame and / or mattress cannot slide away from the wall (a mattress without a frame on a wood or otherwise slippery floor will not work, and neither will a futon).
> Your bed or mattress is against a wall free of heating units or (if you have a futon) the frame is close to the floor and is not against a wall on either side
> Pillows are tightly shoved between the wall and the mattress to prevent a gap
> The baby sleeps next to the wall rather than the edge
> There is a safe waterproof pad beneath the baby (to protect your own mattress)
> The baby is blanketed in his own bedding rather than in yours

You *will* eventually need a good, safe, easily pack-able and portable **playpen** for reasons too numerous to mention, which can be also used as a sleeping place. Although you may not need it right away, it is best to get one of these before the baby comes, as shopping for large things is a major pain in the neck when you're juggling merchandise with a baby.

A Place for the Baby to Bathe: After trying out several methods, I found that a small plastic tub is your best bet, and can be acquired for next to nothing at a second-hand store or superstore. Although the kitchen sink will work as well, it takes great coordination in order to safely bathe your baby in the kitchen sink, and will not be worth saving the two or three dollars. If you must bathe the baby in the kitchen sink, be sure to:

> Put a towel down in the sink to prevent your infant from sliding around
> Turn the faucet nozzle away while the infant is in the sink
> Have all supplies within reach
> Keep one hand on the baby at all times, support newborn baby's head

Car Seat: Even if you don't have a car, you need a car seat for the infant to ride in any automobile. If you don't have your own car, it is wise to get a car seat that attaches onto a stroller as well because you may have to lug all pieces with you whenever you leave the car, and that can be awkward. Always remember to take the base of the car seat with you when you are finished for the day, as the seat can't be used properly in a car without it.

Unless you are *extremely* comfortable and skilled with your soft infant carrier, the first car seat you own should be the type that you can detach from its base so you can carry the whole seat with you. These seats are heavy and difficult to carry, but to use one of these is what's safest for your baby. Along with your car seat, purchase an **Infant**

Head Support. An infant head support is invaluable to a single mother struggling with the task of transporting the car seat to the car (it may be an understandably bumpy ride), and will be useful during your baby's early days in the stroller as well.

Thermometer: You will most likely receive a digital thermometer from the hospital, but if not, you can probably get one at your local supermarket in the baby supplies aisle.

Nasal Aspirator (that weird little suction device that gets the boogers out of your baby's nose): This too will most likely be acquired during your hospital stay. If not, check the baby aisle in the supermarket.

Receiving Blankets: You will probably need about least six of these, as babies rapidly soil them with spit-ups and diaper failures. If you live in a cold climate, you will also need receiving blankets to drape over the baby's face when he or she is outside in freezing temperatures, as a baby's skin is very sensitive to the cold.

Onesies: If you don't know what a onesie is, you will not find the word in the dictionary, but a onesie is basically a one-piece set of baby underwear, most often with short sleeves, that holds the diaper in place. You must also have *at least* six of these, as they too will possibly be soiled several times in a day.

Stroller / Pram: This is one thing you will not be able to live without, and of all people, a single mother should spare no expense when seeking a quality stroller that best meets her needs. There are four basic types of strollers, and depending on your lifestyle, you might even need one of each! Always make sure that your stroller comes with a guarantee and an option to return it. This is a very important purchase, and you can't afford to screw it up.

The first and most modern type is the **Car Seat/ Stroller**. This might be the stroller you choose if you do a lot of traveling by car and little traveling on foot. With this type of stroller, you detach the car seat from its fixture in the car and affix it to a stroller frame. These contraptions are convenient, safe, and are excellent for newborns, but should be regarded as a temporary convenience, as my son outgrew his Car Seat/ Stroller seat by the time he was six months old. Also, by the time your child likes to wiggle around a little, this type of stroller will make him feel very confined.

The second and most common type is the **convertible stroller.** This type of stroller is padded and comfortable, can seat the baby upright or provide an area for him to lie down, and provides storage for the things you need to lug around under the baby's seat. These strollers are good for all-day urban or suburban outings, shopping, long walks through parks with sidewalks and grass, and some errand running. The quilted lining tends to make mothers more secure about their baby's comfort, especially if they live in cold climates. These strollers are generally rather expensive, roughly between eighty and two hundred dollars. Although decent ones can often be found second-hand, look at new ones as well, as the difference in price may be worth having the instructions, warranty, and product demonstration. Always familiarize yourself with all features: brakes, wheels, adjustable handles, etc. before you buy anything.

The third type is the **umbrella stroller**. Although umbrella strollers normally don't have the storage space that the convertibles have, they are extremely light, convenient, and versatile, are very appropriate for travel by air, by city bus, by train, or if you live in a very crowded urban area. A few things you can do with an umbrella stroller that you can't do with a convertible stroller is take it on an escalator (by tipping the front wheels up and balancing the bottom wheels on a stair), up and down stairs, and in narrow hallways. In addition, you can expect to use your umbrella stroller until your child is a toddler. Unlike the convertible stroller, umbrella strollers vary greatly in price, but they also vary greatly in quality. Although some can be obtained for as little as six dollars, some will cost you up to five hundred dollars! True, I have been nagging you about pinching your pennies, but as far as umbrella strollers are concerned, you are better off getting a good one. Depending on where you live, a really good umbrella stroller might be the only stroller you need! Many urbanites like to supplement the use of their umbrella stroller with that of a soft carrier. This combination renders you nearly invincible if you are certain that you will not come upon the opportunity to ride in a car.

Questions to ask yourself or your retailer while you're shopping for an umbrella stroller:

> *How soon can I start to use it and for how long?* If you are going to spend a bundle, make sure your stroller can be used from infancy to toddlerhood.
>
> *If I put a lot of weight on it, does it cause the wheels to stick?* The better the stroller, the better the wheels will be. Check the wheels out really well.
>
> *Does it provide a nice, smooth ride?* This is not only for the benefit of the baby. The less work you have to do, the happier you will be.
>
> *Can I carry it with one hand if I have to?* Everyone has her own opinion of what's too heavy. Gauge your priorities and decide for yourself.
>
> *Is it easy to fold up?* You can't afford to have to wrestle with something.
>
> *Is there enough growing room for my baby?* My first umbrella stroller (there were many, which is why it is important to get one that will last) was too narrow to fit my son's hips when he was merely nine months old. Don't let this happen to you!
>
> *When it is completely folded up, are there sharp metal pieces that stick out and can injure me or my baby? And can all such pieces be secured?* In the case of my old and cheap umbrella stroller, the answer was no, but

I carried around a bungee cord to hold it all together when I had to transport it all packed up.

Do I have to bend over in order to reach the handles? Minimize the stress on your body—it has been through enough with childbirth. Minimize your having to carry things that are too heavy and relying too much on your stronger side. The handles should adjust to your height.

The Fourth Type is the **Jogger**, those strollers that are intended for jogging and other outdoor activities. Joggers are a necessity for outdoorsy people, and like the umbrella stroller, you might be using it until your child is four or even five! These, just like the umbrella strollers, can be very expensive. However, I have found good ones for less than one hundred dollars. The main features you want to look for are these:

That the wheels provide a smooth ride, even when lots of weight is put on them
That the stroller itself is *light* and *easy to push*
That the tread on the tires is designed not to pick up mud
It's easy to fold for transport or storage

If you can only afford one stroller right now, read over these descriptions, evaluate your lifestyle and what's going to be most convenient for you, and start with whichever one you need first. As one who went through *six* strollers during her child's infancy (my big mistake was constantly going for cheapest), take it from me: You're better off getting something top-of-the line than you are if you're constantly having to replace equipment or finding out the hard way why it was so inexpensive. When you're done with higher end equipment, if it's still in good condition, you can get good money for it at the second-hand store.

You also must have a good supply of **non-disposable or cloth diapers.** Regardless of whether you're going for cloth or disposables, you should have a supply of both.

If you have decided to go green and buy cloth, make sure you have some disposables on hand too, because you never know when you're going to be too exhausted to bother with laundering the cloth diapers, and the fact remains that disposables are better for when you're out of the house, and are necessary for when you child is in day care.

If you have decided to use disposables, keep some cloth ones as well. You might wake up in the middle of the night to change the baby and be surprised to find that the diaper bag that you thought was full was just full of air, creating the illusion that you had many more diapers than you really had.

Waterproof Pads: It is necessary to have a couple of waterproof pads to place under the baby while he or she sleeps (especially when the baby is sleeping in YOUR bed), but they must be intended for use with a baby, otherwise they may not be safe. Waterproof pads are inexpensive and will greatly cut down on the amount of laundry you will have to do. Also be sure to acquire a portable **changing pad** that you can carry with you for when you have to change the baby at a friend's house or in public.

Dirty Duds Bag: This item can be as simple as a large Ziploc bag, and will be used to transport a change of clothing or soiled garments while you are out on the town.

Clothes: What you need in the area of clothes will depend on the climate you live in, but you should have at least five sets of pajamas, two or three outfits for public, and plenty of socks. If you live in a cold climate, it is wise to have a couple of polar fleece suits that come with hoods and cover the baby's hands and feet.

Three Important Books: You must acquire (purchase if you must) three necessary reference books that you will want or need to refer back to numerous times throughout your pregnancy and motherhood:

1. A strictly medical book about your baby's development and your physical changes throughout your pregnancy
2. A book about the safety of baby products
3. A book about caring for an infant and small child (might be obtained from your pediatrician)

Everything else can be borrowed or read through and sold, unless you have specialized needs.

A Baby Monitor: Although a rather expensive item, as a single mother you *will* need a baby monitor to put your mind at ease when you *have* to leave your sleeping little one in the house for a moment while you take out the garbage or check the mailbox, etc. Although you may be judged on occasion for leaving the baby alone for a moment, you really have no choice in the matter, and it might be a little fact of life that you prefer not to share with those around you. Do not depend on the monitor for more than a necessary few moments to get these tasks completed. There have been tragic events when people relied on baby monitors for more than a brief time, so don't let this happen to you. It is wise to affix a key chain and extra house key to your baby monitor to ensure that you don't get locked out of your house with the baby inside.

A Breastfeeding Pillow (even if you don't plan to breastfeed): Having a Breastfeeding pillow will really save your back (and those of your friends and relatives) while you are holding your baby, even if you don't plan to breastfeed.

♦ ♦ ♦

Your Checklist

A place for the baby to sleep
Portable playpen
A place for the baby to bathe
Car seat & infant head support
Digital thermometer
Nasal aspirator
Six receiving blankets
Six onesies
Bottles & formula
Stroller
Diapers
Waterproof pads
Portable changing pad
Dirty duds bag
Clothes
Three important books
Baby monitor
Breastfeeding pillow

Chapter Nine

Your Living Space

Deciding if you have the right living space to live comfortably with a baby is of utmost importance. When we address this issue, we need to look at three important components: quantity of space (is there enough of it), quality of space (cleanliness, manageability, and safety), and the location of where you live, which includes how near or far it is from other places you want to get to.

The issue of your living arrangements is something deserves some serious thought *and* action. It's a part of your life needs to be made right *before* your baby is born, and it is likely to be an area in your life that requires you to make some significant changes, even if you choose to remain in the same place. Additionally, it is wise to choose a place that will keep you happy for about three years, because relocating with a baby or toddler can be an overwhelming and exhausting task. At the very least, do not plan to move—unless you're in a bad situation—less than three months before your approximate due date, or in the first six months after birth, as moving at these times can be extremely stressful.

Before any action is taken, ask yourself these questions:

About the Physical Space: Do I have enough space for the baby in the place where I presently live? Do I have enough space to store diapers, clothes, strollers, and other equipment while providing a safe and clean environment for me and for the baby?

Live-In Family or Roommates: Will my having a baby cause any problems with the other people in my household? Should I try to work through these potential problems, or are we better off moving out, or asking them to move out now (if you hold the lease or own the home)?

Financial Concerns: Can I afford to stay where I am? Should I rent or buy?

A Satisfying Life: Am I completely happy with where I live? Do I have important friends and family in this area? Can I maintain a social life here? Can I get/do I have the right kind of job/ growth opportunities and the right kind of child care?

Quantity of Space—How much is enough for you?

This is a good time to revisit the idea of what kind of person you are when it comes to how much space you need in order to fully enjoy your domestic life with a baby. For example, you may be the type of person who likes to have control over her home, likes to know exactly where things are, and likes to be able to do what she wants when she wants without having to worry about anyone else's schedule or priorities. You may enjoy having your mother or friends over for extended periods of time, but may also appreciate the silence after they've gone home, as well as the opportunity to get back into your routine. For you, having a roommate or living with others in anything but a large space may compromise your quality of life.

On the other hand, you may be the type of person who thrives in an atmosphere of community. You may be accustomed to sharing your space with roommates and guests, and having people around may help you to be relaxed. Dishes in the sink don't bother you much, and a constant source of background noise such as a TV or radio makes you feel right at home. You can fall asleep easily on an airplane or at a friend's house. For these kind of women, living alone with a baby is a recipe for depression or worse. If you feel the same way, definitely do not endeavor to strike out on your own at this time in your life!

In my opinion, however, any woman with a baby needs to have a friend or family member whom they can call at any time day or night in case of an emergency. I also feel that every new mother needs a friend or relative to stay with her and help within the first six weeks of the baby's life, as the transition to motherhood can be extremely rocky at times. Even happily married or otherwise well-supported mothers have meltdowns sometimes. Although it happens often enough that it's considered a normal occurrence, it is a clear sign that one needs help immediately. It is for this reason that I strongly recommend having enough space to accommodate overnight guests (see following paragraphs on living alone). Also, if you choose to live alone, do invest some time and energy into building your support community, and make a list of those people you can call in the event that you feel like you're going to lose control.

For Those Who Choose to Live Alone

If you live in a city or town where housing prices are out of control, you'll be pleased to know that I have found a **one bedroom apartment or condo to be an ideal residence for a single mother with a baby**. Not only is it easier to make your rent or mortgage payments than if you had a larger place, but it's also easier to stay organized and refrain from doing any unnecessary spending or accumulating useless items because of your limited space. In the event that your baby has been crying for twenty minutes and you need to put a closed door between the two of you while you catch your breath, it's easily done. If, on the other hand, you want to be nearby to hear the baby when they wake up, there you are.

If you decide to live in a one-bedroom apartment or condo, the organization of your house will be simple: The bedroom can be for sleeping and dressing, and the living room can be for working, watching TV, visiting, or anything else that requires activity. This way, if you have friends over or have work to do, you can tend to your noisier tasks while the baby sleeps in another room, separated from all the action. If you go this route, you will be wise to acquire a double convertible or futon sofa or a couch large enough to sleep on for your living room. This can serve as a crashing place for visiting friends or family (sometimes when you have a baby your social life is limited to those who will come see you), and will be an alternate place to sleep in the event that you are tossing and turning, or if you just need some space to yourself.

However, I have found that keeping a baby alone in an **efficiency** or **studio apartment** can be a challenge. Your schedule will have to revolve 100 percent around your baby's schedule, and the absence of compartmentalized space (separate rooms with doors that close) may provide challenges in keeping organized, having the freedom to do whatever you want while the baby sleeps, and maintaining a social or romantic life in your home.

When my son was little, he wanted my full attention at every waking moment. But when he was napping, I had a two-hour window to rush around and do dishes, vacuum, listen to music, dance, practice my violin, visit with friends, start cooking a great meal for myself, or take part in any other activity that might have disturbed him. If I hadn't used this short amount of time to get my house clean and straight, I feel that I might have gone crazy, as not only do I thrive in an organized atmosphere, but when I clean, cook, read, meditate, or practice my instruments, I like to focus deeply on what I'm doing. I found that by the time my son awoke and my "recess" was over, I usually felt as though I'd had enough "me time" to give my child my full attention once more.

For some people, having this break of being able to deeply focus on something is as important as sleep is for others. When you have a baby, so much of your life belongs to your child. Your child will often require your full attention when he is awake, but if he's asleep and you have two separate rooms, your life can be yours once again, if only for a couple of hours.

In my opinion, if you don't currently live in a rent-controlled or otherwise inexpensive studio with at least a large closet or reading room/dining room nook, you shouldn't move into one unless every other option seems worse (bad roommates, too expensive, etc.).

Living alone in a **house** or **apartment with more than one bedroom** can be perceived as a luxury worth seeking by some single mothers, but others find that having too much space provides too much opportunity to become disorganized. For example, an extra bedroom can become the place where unfolded laundry and other things just pile up. Just as too much time in each other's faces can be nerve-wracking, too much physical space between a mother and her baby can be a stress. If you already live in an apartment with two or more bedrooms, your payments are manageable, and the place has become home to you, it's not necessary to downgrade in order to conform to the advice I give here. However, if you are currently happy in a one-bedroom apartment or condo, don't feel like you need to have more than one bedroom in order to provide your child with everything that's needed.

For Those Who Prefer to Live With Others:
If you live with roommates or your family, just make sure that you have at least one bedroom to yourself and your baby. Most mothers get more restful sleep when their baby is in the room with them. In addition, you can respond to your baby's needs almost instantly, and if you breastfeed, you will probably become good at feeding in the night without fully waking up.

Having two bedrooms to yourself in a roommate situation might be the ideal, because you can use one bedroom for sleeping, and the other as an extra bedroom, an activity room, or private living room for you and the baby, or as an alternate place to do whatever you like at the odd hours that you will be awake. This way you can control the safety and cleanliness of the room without compromising the priorities of your roommates, and you won't make waves if too much baby gear accumulates here. It often does not matter how large the rooms are, and some folks have successfully placed a bed in a walk-in closet as a makeshift bedroom.

The Quality of Your Space
Wherever you are, the key to making your living arrangement work requires two simple (but not always easy) things. First, eliminate clutter. Second, stay organized. The key is not having many things in the first place and loving the few things you have. Soon you will naturally be accumulating more stuff, whether you buy it or it's given to you. If you have things you are pretty sure you will want or need during the first six months after birth, you'll need enough room to stow it away while having easy access to it.

If you are reading this in the early stage of your pregnancy, this is the time to begin the process of paring down the things in your life, while you're mobile and agile.

Clutter, and What to do With it…
A good project to get started on is eliminating everything you are not madly in love with or are not certain that you will need between now and six months after birth (refer back to **Chapter 5**). Have a garage sale or tag sale. Mark the prices low so your stuff will move. Also think about what you have that might fetch a good price on Craiglist.org or an online auction site: Designer clothes, rare recordings, art, ceramics, perfume, and other expensive or even unusual items (especially good brand names). Take the nicer clothes you

haven't worn for years to a consignment store that will either pay you cash or give you money in trade for products they have. Likewise, you can take books, videos, and other items to a second-hand store that will let you sell or get trade credit (or a lower amount of cash) for them. Put ads on bulletin boards. Ask your friends if they'd be interested in taking anything off your hands for a reasonable price. Get rid of knick-knacks that don't have any deep sentimental value to you.

For your own peace of mind later, don't be afraid to give or throw things away, especially anything broken, or with holes in them or stains on them. Go through the depths of your kitchen cupboards as well, as that's where you've probably stored a lot of things you don't really use. In terms of food you've been storing, take an inventory of what you have back there, and resolve to use it up. Of course, throw away anything that you feel isn't safe or is past its due date. If you're certain that you are not going to use something, donate it and save the receipt to write off your taxes.

After you've narrowed down what's important and what's not, invest in some organizational aides for your home, especially your closet. A shoe caddy or chest will free up lots of space, and shelves can always be put to good use. Pack up the important things you won't be using for a while and put them on the high shelves in your closets, as you'll need the more accessible space for the baby's things. Make sure you get a good, steady (preferably folding) step stool so you don't have any accidents while you're putting things up and taking them down. This stepstool, by the way, will also eventually become your child's favorite household play toy, opening up the world to a child able to climb. Don't pack those boxes any heavier than ten pounds. Put up an extra bar for hanging the baby's clothes on. Put hooks everywhere you can, because you can hang umbrellas, jackets, hats, purses with straps, shopping bags and lots more, keeping them off the floor or off of shelf space that can be used for other things.

Promise yourself that you will use up all those lotions, soaps, and shampoo samples you've acquired that have been piling up in your cabinets and drawers. Throw away those old tubes of mascara, out-of-date lipsticks, and stale perfumes. If something is still good, use it up. Make sure everything has its proper place, and that it's not just hanging out on the bathroom counter or the kitchen table.

Whether or not you will actually need any bedroom furniture for your baby is a personal decision based on your comfort and budget. Throughout history, babies generally never had their own furniture until door-to-door salesmen started targeting working class neighborhoods, trying to sell baby furniture to people who had much more important things to do with their money, which resulted in many people thinking that baby furniture is a necessity for the mother who wants to give her child the best of everything. But based on my experience and research of a mother's comfort and a baby's needs, giving your baby the best of everything has nothing to do with providing several pieces of furniture. All around the world mothers create spaces for themselves and their babies without big pieces of furniture. In some parts of the world, mothers and babies sleep in a hammock slung low to the floor. In other parts of the world, the whole family shares a bed, which is not regarded as the site to engage in intimate sexual activity, but is rather the place where everyone sleeps. Although these facts might not mesh with your preferred lifestyle, you get the point: Baby furniture may very well be a waste of your money and space.

When you have a baby, make sure your house is a shoes-off atmosphere. In many parts of the world where both space and furniture in homes are kept to a minimum, no one would think of wearing outdoor shoes inside the house. For one thing, babies are often safer on the floor than on furniture. Even if it's not a normal practice where you live, it is a good idea to make your home a "shoes off" home, at least while your baby spends time exploring the floor.

If you don't already have a designated place for shoes, you can find a rolling storage cart at your local superstore. If you have to clean under it, temporarily move it into a closet, it's easily done. A place for shoes, boots and other outside clothing by the door is a good idea, along with a place to hang outdoor clothes. That might be where you also park a wheeled push-pull cart that you can use both for food shopping or for taking clothes to the laundry in the event that you don't have a washer and drying or clothes line on the premises.

It is recommended that your baby's clothes are kept hung in a closet or in drawers rather than out in the open, as unnecessary exposure to dust may contribute to respiratory problems for some babies, and insects and other pests can more easily access things in open containers. Thus, you will need a place to store your baby's clothes, but that might be in a couple of drawers in the dresser you already have. I found that my son's clothes all fit into two drawers in my own dresser for the first couple of years of his life. You can also acquire an inexpensive small plastic set of drawers at a superstore.

Other ideas for creating more space: depending on the climate in which you live or other potentially limiting factors, you may consider having a large mattress or large futon as your bed, rather than one up high on a frame, with a box spring. Your baby can sleep alongside you, either in the bed, or on a little mattress right next to your bed, and be perfectly safe, so long as you take the necessary precautions.

For example, if you don't have an extremely heavy and firm mattress, don't have the side of the mattress where the baby is up against a wall, because that can be a place where a baby can wedge himself in the crack, and don't try this at all if you have a hardwood, tile, laminate, or linoleum floor, as even a firm and heavy mattress can slide (only attempt this sleeping arrangement with a very firm mattress upon a carpeted floor). Babies have been badly injured, or worse, by being wedged against the wall when the appropriate cautions have not been observed. If you can't wedge your arm between the mattress and the wall without physically dragging the mattress away from the wall, it is likely firm and heavy enough. If you do have a firm mattress combined with a heavy enough bed frame that would never think of sliding away from the wall (like I did), you can push the bed alongside the wall and wedge sofa pillows or throw pillows between the mattress and the wall & headboard. Also, make sure that any wall and floor that border your mattress are free of heating or air conditioning units.

A quick interjection on mattresses: Don't ever consider purchasing or acquiring what is known as a "rebuilt" or "reconditioned" mattress or box springs in order to save money, as the padding is often assembled around components of an old mattress that can (and often do) harbor mold, insects, and toxins that can be extremely hazardous to the health of the people sleeping there. Thankfully, the law states that a rebuilt mattress must be presented as such, but salespeople often attempt to downplay their potential hazards. If you are in the market for an inexpensive mattress, you are far better off getting a futon or even an air mattress than what is known as a "re-built" mattress.

In your common areas, do consider what you need and what you truly love versus what you have simply grown accustomed to, and make adjustments depending on your priorities. Watch for safety issues: Sharp edges can be dangerous to both you and the baby, plant stands or other items that tip over easily can be treacherous, etc. Consider hanging the plants instead. Consider installing a sturdy shelf (make sure you use the anchors) and getting rid of (or stash away) the end table with the wobbly leg. If you love something, make it work, but know that your love for an item might change when you find that you have to sprint across the room every time the baby goes near it.

When you've done all the dreaming, planning, and adjusting that you can, it's a good time to ask yourself one final time, "Do I have enough space?" If the answer is still "no," then a move might be in order, and it's much better that it be done sooner than later. Aren't you glad everything is packed up so neatly?

Roommates/People
If You Live on Someone Else's "Turf"
If you feel that living with other people is best for your emotional and physical needs, feel out your situation and make sure it's right. Before the baby arrives is the best time for everyone to clarify needs and wishes and make a set of agreements for what each person is responsible for or expected to do—or not do. Do everything you can to make the relationships with the people who are most important to you be as good as they can be, and never take a loved one for granted. After the birth, it becomes much more difficult for you to work around other people's needs—or even think about them, much less put them first. Make sure that your communication is clear before the birth of your child.

Family

If your parents or other close relatives offer free room and board, it is usually a good idea to accept that help, especially in the first months right after birth. Just be as certain as possible that your presence will not earn you any pressure, criticism, or emotional abuse. If you do take the charity of your family, save your money as diligently as though you were paying rent. Sometimes the gravy train unexpectedly jumps the tracks, and sometimes a woman comes to the conclusion that living with parents or other relatives is far more difficult than striking out on their own. This, of course, varies widely from case to case.

Living with family can sometimes compromise your ability to have a social life, even just a friend over to watch a movie. Talk about this ahead of moving in and find out what the expectations are and discuss your desires and see how they mesh. Honest verbal communication so often prevents angry upsets after small things build up to a blowing point. Make sure any issues are addressed before they become problems.

Roommates

Living with other people can be a great way to have ready access to your social life while going through a potentially isolating season in your life. If your roommates are mature, stable, loving, and are consistent parts of your life, they might welcome your baby into your shared home and your family of friends. However, living with roommates can also be difficult unless your roommates are extremely understanding about babies crying all night and the equipment that will inevitably expand into common areas, as well as keeping shared space organized and safe. It must be mentioned that sometimes even the best of friends (roommates, parents, partners, etc.) run screaming when they are not ready for a baby to enter the picture. Babies can cause all sorts of disruptions that can throw lives into disarray. If you do plan to remain with your roommates, make sure they are prepared for life to change, and ask yourself *and any roommates/housemates you are going to have,* these questions:

Can my roommates live with a baby? Warn your roommates that sometimes there will be nothing you can do about your crying baby, the fact that your stroller was left in the hallway because you had to get to work quickly, the house smelling faintly of diapers, and the fact that you had to sleep on the couch that night. Assure them that you will do your best, but let them know that if any of this is going to significantly strain your relationship, you need to know NOW.

Can I have the bedroom that is farthest away from the other bedrooms? If one of the bedrooms is separated from the others, this is the one you should have, at least for now. If this bedroom costs more than the others, then go ahead and shell out the bucks to get this better place. Even if there are a few grumbles in the house, after a night of hearing the baby cry, your roommates will be glad that the baby is far away rather than right next to them.

Are my roommates too messy, careless, or unsafe to have around my baby? I had what I thought was a great roommate when my son was about nine months old. She was loving, patient, and accommodating. But despite all her good characteristics, she had a stormy relationship with her boyfriend, and one time I even found that she had spilled some of her medication on the floor and hadn't gotten it completely cleaned up before she left for work. She was a good friend and paid her rent on time, but yelling boyfriends and pills on the floor are things a mother with a baby just can't live with.

Have you ever seen your roommates act in a way that you perceive as violent, dangerous, unreasonable, extremely insensitive, or otherwise dysfunctional? Does anyone you plan to live with smoke in the house? Do they ever have "shady" houseguests? Does anyone play their music too loud for you? After you have a baby, you'll be surprised at your intolerance for things you used to have no problem with.

If you are now feeling (or have been subtly informed) that your roommates can't handle a baby in the household but you don't have enough money to go it on your own, you might try looking for another single mother to live with. You may be able to work opposite hours and even eliminate both the cost of child care and the challenge of finding a babysitter. You can also share household responsibilities cook together or cook on different nights, so that you can each have some dinners that you don't have to prepare. Besides that you can trade off babysitting for each other, to give you each a few hours on your own. Whatever you decide to do, make sure you screen people *thoroughly* for financial stability as well as emotional stability, and also for lifestyle, personality, and cleanliness (and personal habits, like smoking, drinking, going to bed very late or very early…) before you move in with them.

There is a nonprofit called coabode (coabode.org) that helps single mothers by finding them living situations with other single mothers for the benefits of those reasons listed above and others. My impression is that they have a large network, as plugging in the zip code of my small town yielded 67 potential roommates. If you don't have a roommate situation that you are sold on, this is a resource to look into.

What Can I Afford?

Depending on your lifestyle, you may have been comfortable spending half of your income or more on your housing, but as a former mortgage industry professional, I know that this is generally a bad idea, *especially* when a baby is on the way. For one thing, babies tend to come with lots of extra expenses, both expected (possible day care, health or medical costs), and unexpected. If you are spending more than *one third* of your gross income on housing, you may want to consider moving.

Your Quality of Life
Certain things we are accustomed to when you are mobile and free can be a major pain in the neck when you have a baby. Such things include, but are not limited to:

Security Entrances:
Although, in theory, security entrances are good things, imagine trying to juggle keys, groceries, *and* your baby, while staying out of the way of a heavy iron door with sharp edges. It can be tricky and very frustrating when you have to do it day after day. As for the keys to your entrance, you may be able to minimize stress by entrusting a neighbor or apartment manager to a set of your keys in the event that something –or someone –gets locked in or locked out.

Too Many Stairs:
Again, stairs are good and bad at the same time. Steep, sharp, slippery, and hard stairs can be treacherous. Climbing stairs with a baby in your arms (or in a sling or soft baby carrier) is a fantastic workout, but it can really do a number on your attitude, especially if you're also trying to carry up groceries or a stroller, etc.

Parking Issues:
Do you have to move your car every other day in order to give clearance for the street cleaners or on snow removal days? Hiking home from a parking spot is great exercise when you don't have a baby, but not much fun when you have to do it with your baby, especially if she's hungry or tired and complaining, or you're both cranky.

When I lived in San Francisco, I sometimes had to drive for a half-hour to find a parking space to avoid a parking ticket, and sometimes I had to walk a half mile back to my apartment. If this sounds like something you have to do, really consider whether or not you need the car at all, or whether you'd be better off living in a suburb or an apartment that provides parking.

Distance from conveniences:
If you live in a city, you will probably want to be within easy walking distance of a market that's open late or early, maybe a bank or place you can withdraw money from a machine, and a trusted babysitter or childcare facility. If you are not living in a city, especially if you are living pretty far from other mothers and babies or helpful friends or family members, you will have to stay organized in order to keep your place stocked with the things you will need.

Nature, parks and other beautiful places

It is important for you and the baby to get out into the world and watch life happening around you. Even if the weather is not excellent, babies, toddlers, children, and adults benefit from seeing dogs, butterflies, flowers, grass, and other people. You might not get to the park every day or even every week, but you'll be glad it's there when you want it, especially when you child becomes interested in playgrounds, or if your mood can be vastly improved by being in nature. Think of the nearby out-of-doors as an extension of the place where you and your baby live, because it can make life a whole lot less stressful on a new mom to be able to walk or take a bus to a beautiful place that both you and your baby enjoy.

If you live in a city, you might think about any museums that you would like to be able to access easily. Some children's museums, science museums, or museums with children's areas have affordable memberships that enable a parent to go often without paying for entry every time they go. Memberships such as these can be especially helpful for those who live in extremely cold or hot climates.

Other Things that Make Life Easier

Regardless of the possible drawbacks of your living situation, if you have ready access to certain conveniences, you are in a good place to live with a baby. Take note of how far the following conveniences are from where you currently live. If you decide to move, make sure you note your distance from these conveniences and consider their importance to you before you sign any lease.

24-Hour Emergency Clinic:

Sure, you'll never need it if it's nearby. However, if you're living on your own and especially if you tend to be the worrying type, it's not a bad idea. Cheat Murphy's Law by making sure an emergency clinic is close at hand.

Your Job

Think of how nice it will be when your boss lets you off work early on a sunny day, and you can accept a co-worker's invitation to have a cup of tea or coffee before you pick the baby up. More than that, think how nice it would be to have a childcare place or person within a few minutes' walk from where you work so that you can take time off once every couple of hours to go be with your baby. Having babysitter, home, and job all in the same area can definitely de-complicate your life!

Bank Branch or No-fee Automated Teller Machine

While most people these days are paying with plastic, there will be some times that you need cash or need to deposit a physical check immediately. It might really make you mad if you have to pay two dollars to access your own money. Some banks and credit unions still have night drops for checks—I admit I have been relieved when I knew I could stay one step ahead of an overdraft by putting a check in the night drop at ten o'clock at night. If your bank provides the ability to deposit checks with your smartphone, learn how to do that.

Corner Store
Again, think of all the possibilities of what can happen in the middle of the night, or after an exhausting day of caring for your baby and needing to get some work done too. You need access to food, diapers, batteries, and possibly formula (remember that organic is best if you use formula) without having to go through a huge ordeal to get it.

Parking
If you own a car, you won't want to park it on the street and have to move it every other day for the street cleaners—and you don't need a $20 ticket because you didn't want to wake a peacefully sleeping baby to get this done. If your car is necessary and the place you are living doesn't have parking, make plans to move as soon as you can. If you have considered renting such a place, pass on the opportunity for the time being.

Trusted Day Care Facility or Babysitter
You don't want to have to drive your car or take busses or subways all over town just to take your baby to a place where he is going to be safe and loved and nurtured for a few hours. Having everything as close by as possible will make life much easier, calmer and happier, for your baby as well as for you. Remember, the goal is to find a way to lead a *low-stress* life with your baby. These are the months that lay down the patterns in your baby's nervous system and brain for the rest of life. And they also set patterns of tension or ease in your *own* life!

Laundromat or on-site laundry facilities
Whether you live in a rural area, a town, or in a city, it is a huge challenge to safely haul laundry and a baby at the same time. Depending on where you live, there might be social benefits of going to your particular local Laundromat (especially if it has some a coffee shop, second hand store, market, or library a few doors away). However, consider that leaving your home to get *anything* done is usually going to take away time you could spend doing something more fun and productive. When I lived in San Francisco, I was lucky to have a laundry "wash-and-fold" service right downstairs—and it was affordable. If you have such conveniences in your area, find out where they are and how much it

costs to have someone else wash, dry and fold your laundry for you. Also realize that, despite our modern standards, dryers are never necessary, as if you don't have access to a clothesline, a portable drying rack will certainly do the trick (I personally never saw one until I lived in Europe, where they're the norm), but to air-dry certain clothes might result in having to iron them, which for many people is a most unpleasant chore, especially when trying to care for a baby.

Post Office
The act of mailing a package should not be an all-day chore, but that's what it can be if your post office is not easily accessible. The idea of making a mistake with an online purchase used to fill me with frustration and fear—between work and child care, when was I going to have time to get to the post office? Sometimes I'd be stuck with a purchase that wasn't right simply because I could not fit a trip to the post office into my schedule. Later in my professional life, when I was working for a company that moved into a mall with a post office, I could get an errand like this done on a fifteen-minute break, which was a huge relief. I started dressing better, returns were less stressful, and I got better at sending gifts and cards on time as well.

Being near a post office may be of less importance to those who can send purchases to their office, or those who can use office postage scales to calculate postage, etc. For those new to the world of office work, be sure to ask your supervisor if you ever plan to use stationery. Taking even little things without asking can put an employee in the hot seat.

Some other features that might tip the scales when evaluating your living situation are:

Rent Control
If your rent is guaranteed never to go up, especially in an urban or densely populated area, hang on for dear life and save like there's no tomorrow. A friend of mine in San Francisco pays $600.00 a month for a studio apartment with an oversized walk-in closet (half the size of her living/bedroom) with doors and a very small dining room that she can close off. New renters are spending in the ballpark of $2500 for similar units in the same building. If I had a baby in that place, I would find a way to make it work until I just couldn't take it anymore.

Outdoor Common Area/ Courtyard
Sometimes a little sunshine, some grass, and a nice bench to sit on are all you need to get grounded when a walk down the street to a public area is more than you want to commit to.

Sustainability

What are the physical features of this house or apartment (yard, woodstove, greenhouse, balcony, windows, access to public transport, proximity to food market) that can help decrease your dependency on gas, energy, and grocery stores? Being at least somewhat self-sufficient can be a real blessing for anyone: Doubly so for a mother with an infant.

Other elements you might want to figure into your scenario include:

> ***Church, synagogue, or other spiritual center***
> ***Gym:*** You will appreciate being close to a baby-friendly gym with a heated, preferably saline (rather than chlorinated) pool, because swimming or just being with your baby in warm water is a great way for both of you to relax, exercise, and enjoy life together. Research the facility to assure that babies are allowed in the pool on your schedule before you invest in a membership. Some gyms also provide short-term day care, which should be looked into, but often have age limits for the children they take.
> ***Yoga, dance, or tai chi studio:*** Some yoga classes are specifically for mothers with babies. Others studios have childcare on site or a few doors away.
> ***Restaurant, café, coffee shop or natural food store with a deli***
> ***Friends and family***
> ***A clean pub or tavern with "non-creepy" staff and clientele:*** If you can people watch, converse, and have a glass of wine in public with a girlfriend without getting harassed every five minutes, it's great to have a place to do so nearby. On the other hand, noisy club-type bars are never pleasant neighbors.

Creating Your Own Personal Recipe for Happiness

Do you *like* living in your city or town, or are you just *used to* living where you live? In your town, do you have access to the activities you enjoy, the kind of people you want to meet, and the job that you have always dreamed of? If the answer is no, then what is keeping you there? Is it your family? Is it your job, or fear of the unknown?

It's true that moving to a different city or state right before you have a baby is a bit reckless unless you have special reasons to get out of the town or state where you live— but for the rest of you, why not at least work towards getting exactly what we want out of life? Just as in everything else right now, your progress may appear to be slow for a couple of years, but if you find an opportunity that is absolutely right for you, don't fail to take it simply because it seemed to happen too fast. There is a great diversity in our destinies and how you find it. No two stories are the same.

Evaluate those activities that do bring you joy, and make adjustments to include those activities in your life. Is skiing your favorite activity? If you've always wanted to live in a ski resort town, start doing research. You might even find your dream job, an apartment, and a babysitter on line, bringing you right to the life you've always dreamed of.

Are you a live music addict, or a person who would like to live in a place warm enough to wear shorts during all four seasons? Do you crave the "action" and artistic savvy of the city? Or, do you feel you might be most at peace and happy living in a small cabin in the woods while you tend to your organic garden?

Pinpoint your dreams, and go after them. Don't let our society tell you that your life is over because you're about to be a mother. Your only situation you really need to commit to is taking the best care of your child while you live your own life to the fullest.

If A Move is In Order...
If, after all your evaluating, you find that a move is in order, try to do so in your first or second trimester, and avoid heavy lifting at all costs!

Although I'm always urging you to be frugal with your money, I personally am a big fan of professional movers. If you have the money, and if you have any fewer than five strong friends who are enthusiastic about helping you, then—unless your heaviest piece of furniture is a futon frame or a beanbag chair—look for the smallest, most independent moving companies in your area, compare prices, haggle, ask if they will charge you for a whole hour if you only use a half hour, ask if their student or senior citizen discounts might apply to single pregnant women, etc. Professional movers will normally take everything in one trip (but you must have everything boxed up), which will save you *a lot* of time, gasoline, the hassle of parking and re-parking, and will spare you potential for injury. Also, a good professional mover will be careful not to scrape your walls or damage your furniture. They will consider the order that the furniture needs to go in and out of the truck for your unpacking convenience.

If you *do* have a very strong friend or relative who has a big truck, a ton of enthusiasm, and who would like to make a dollar or two helping you out, still call around and find prices for the professionals. You don't want to pay your friend the same amount that is required for a professional, as there are greater risks involved when friends do business. Your friend might damage your furniture, injure him/herself (the professionals are insured if this happens), or decide in the middle of moving that they're not being paid enough for this job. When these things happen, you end up having to hire the professionals anyway.

If you have a whole gaggle of friends or relatives who are going to help you for free, you are a very lucky person. Try to compensate for any free help you receive (I know people who have bribed their friends and sometimes their friends' kids to do anything by offering pizza), and pack all the boxes you plan to carry yourself as lightly as you possibly can.

Remember that moving is an exhausting process—eat healthily throughout your move, drink lots of water, don't let yourself get worn out, get plenty of rest, and (very important) don't put an unreasonable time limit on your transition. If you are not using professional movers, make sure you have access to both your new place and your old place for at least one week. Start taking boxes over to your new place as soon as possible. Plan to have everything moved at least three days before you no longer have access to your old place, as you may need three days to arrange to get your old place cleaned in order to get your deposit back, and you may need a last look around to make sure you didn't leave your coin collection on top of the refrigerator (a friend of mine actually found a valuable collection of coins in a condo he had bought) or your picture of grandma on the shelf of your closet. For those of us who tend to grow roots, this "last look around" can sometimes be an emotional experience, so give yourself time to say goodbye.

Is It Time to Buy?
Although in some parts of the country home ownership is impossible for people who aren't rich, many single people, young people, and lower income people are surprised to find that yes, they can indeed own a home. If you have held steady employment for at least two years (or have been in college or a training program to develop mastery in the field in which you are now working), have good credit, and are certain that you want to stay in the city or town where you live, you might look into the possibility of buying a house or a condo. However, prices, availability, and quality vary widely from city to city and town to town. The only way to find out if you can buy is to go to a mortgage company and get pre-qualified.

Step 1: Pre-qualification at a Bank, Credit Union, or Mortgage Company
Pre-qualification is the method of determining how much house one can afford. Although visiting a loan officer might be intimidating, it will probably be much easier than you think, and the service of pre-qualification does not cost you anything— your loan officer gets paid only after your house has been purchased, and the "Loan Origination Fee," which is split between the loan officer and her company, should only be about 1 percent of your loan amount, which will probably be within one or two thousand dollars of your sales price, depending on the financing you ultimately choose.

The loan officer will ask you questions about your job, how much money you make, where you have lived, and will ask you to bring in documentation showing your income (pay stubs and tax records), your bank statements, and your identity (driver's license, social security card, etc.), and she will run your credit report. When she has all the necessary documentation, she will tell you the price of the house you can afford, the size of the house payment you can expect, and the amount of cash you need in order to close (or finish) the deal. Sometimes these costs can be rolled into the loan, so don't be afraid to let her know if you just don't have that cash.

Things you should know:
In the event that your loan officer works at a large national company, she may have access to special reduced interest rate programs and programs that require no down payment for people with special circumstances or lower incomes. On the other hand, it is often great for your local economy to get your mortgage at a local bank or credit union, and they too might have special offers for you. Talk to a few people before you schedule a real sit-down appointment, and choose what seems best for you.

You are entitled to ask questions. When you make your appointment, let the loan officer know that you are new at this. While in your appointment, if your loan officer can't slow down enough to clearly explain things to you, she doesn't deserve your business. Although some things are hard to understand for anyone who isn't a banker (like the fact that your APR is *not* your interest rate), your loan officer must be patient with you. She works *for* you.

After your loan officer has pre-qualified you, although you might have sudden confidence in your money managing abilities, do not do any unnecessary spending on credit. If you get a high credit card balance or spend a large portion of your savings, the amount you qualify for will change, and can change in-between the time you were pre-qualified and the time that you close on your dream house. If your loan officer tells you not to make any large purchases, she means it!

In the event that your credit is too damaged for the loan officer to pre-qualify you, a good loan officer will tell you what you need to do in order to clean your credit up, and she'll invite you to come back in a year or two and try again. If you like her and feel that she has been fair, informative, and respectful to you, always go back to her: These people work on commission. If not, go to someone else next time.

Your loan officer might tell you that although you can afford a hundred thousand dollar house, you can only afford an eighty thousand dollar condo. This is because she figures your condo dues into the monthly payment you can afford. These condo dues usually pay for garbage removal, lawn care, snow removal, exterior maintenance, and other things you would be paying out of pocket if you own a house. As a single mother who has been through this, I think the condo is often a better deal for someone who is about to have a baby.

Mari Gallion

At the time of the first writing of this book, ARMS (Adjustable Rate Mortgages) were *En Vogue*, and I warned my readers against falling prey to them. At this time, I do not believe that Adjustable Rate Mortgages are still available. If they are, just don't get one. In case you don't know what an ARM is, it is a mortgage in which you interest rate is not fixed. Although your interest rate starts out very low, after a period of time it can "adjust," or change to the current interest rate, which might go through the roof. These could be perceived as a good thing in the event that the property values continue to rise, but guess what? What comes up must come down. At the time of *this* writing, we are seeing the result of those people who based their decision on the continued growth paradigm, the idea that everything: salaries, property values, etc., would continue to grow. How much sense does that make in a world with finite resources?

Whatever you do, do not lie to your loan officer. Most of the sensitive information about your situation can be determined from your pay stubs, bank statements, and credit report, so you normally don't have to give her an exact figure on these things (many people don't even know the answers to these questions). But sometimes she will ask you if you have others earning money in your household, whether you have ever been bankrupt, and other questions that might seem invasive. Remember that these are the bank's questions, not hers. If you sign an application that has false information, this is fraud. Don't put yourself or her in this situation. Telling the truth is for your own good.

If you make a large bank deposit while you are trying to buy a house, it usually has to be explained to the bank. If you got that money because you sold your car, keep documentation of the transaction. If a friend or family member gives you money, it needs to be documented with what's called a "gift letter" (ask your loan officer to explain this process). Big piles of money don't just appear out of nowhere. If you've been saving money in a fire safe box, make sure to put it into your bank at least three months before you do any official business with a bank so they don't question why you have it.

While taking your application, your loan officer will probably ask you about your race. Although this is really weird, don't think your loan officer is discriminating against you, as this is our government's way of making sure she is *not* practicing discrimination. If she is shown to approve loans only to those of one race, she will get in big trouble. Although in banking there is an occasional throwback to the Nazi era, your average loan officer truly wants to take your loan, and does not care what color you are. Otherwise she doesn't get paid. If you really feel she has a problem with you because of your race (or ethnicity, or because you're single, or pregnant, etc.), then by all means go to someone else.

Remember to be nice. If your loan officer tells you that you can't get financing, it is not her personal decision—it is because the bank won't loan you money because you don't meet *the bank's* requirements. In addition, if she foresees that you are going to be difficult or rude to her, she has every right not to handle your loan, as sometimes a commission is not worth taking abuse. Do your best to cooperate with what she asks you to do. If you think she's being unfair, visit another bank before you assume she has a personal problem with you. If you get financing elsewhere, it is her loss, right?

If in your past you have demonstrated wise and grounded financial choices, sometimes financially stable parents, siblings, grandparents, or even friends might be willing to co-sign (vouch for your financial responsibility by agreeing to make your payments in the event that you cannot) with you on a house or a condo. If you get someone to co-sign for you, do your absolute best to hold up your part of the deal by making timely payments and caring for the property, as both your credit and theirs could be ruined if you don't. Also consider that division of property can be as messy and costly as a divorce, so please don't enter into this situation lightly. People who extend you this consideration are showing you deep trust and love. If you can't honestly return these strong sentiments (for example, if this offer is made by a suitor with feelings you don't reciprocate or anyone you privately resent or mistrust), please make your angels proud and turn this offer down. Karmic ties to another person are serious business, and it is in everyone's best interest that you stay spiritually clean.

Beware of the term "creative financing." This is sometimes a code word for "unethical loan officer who will do anything for money." Sometimes a loan officer will tell you that you can buy the house you want, only for you to show up at the closing table to find that you're purchasing an Adjustable Rate Mortgage that is going to jump three percentage points in a year. If you need what's called "creative financing" in order to buy a house, the best thing for you to do is accept that for right now, you just can't afford it, and to save up for the future.

Step 2: Agent or no Agent?

It would be wonderful to say that you are better off buying a house through a real estate agent, but although some of them are honest and helpful, some of them are evil and awful. Some popular agents will spend less time trying to help and educate someone who is in the market for an inexpensive house. Some agents who specialize in lower income customers do so because they can take advantage of what they believe to be "less educated" people. Some agents get a lot of business simply because they are extroverted, friendly, or good looking, and really don't have a clue about what they're doing. The question of whether or not you are better off with an agent depends *entirely* on the agent! You are better off getting a Realtor (an agent who belongs to an association committed to practicing good ethics) but even some of them are terrible. Of course, some of them are wonderful, helpful people who find great satisfaction in earning money through helping people find the home of their dreams. Use your intuition when it comes to dealing with any salespeople, and beware of "fast talk."

And just like the fact that agents can be a blessing or a curse, so can some For Sale by Owner sellers. You might buy a house for a good price only to find that it has termites and is on the brink of falling down. Sometimes the seller doesn't even know about problems in their houses, and sometimes they do. Some people want to do the most honest thing, and some are just out for themselves. The best way to prevent yourself from getting into a bad situation with a For Sale by Owner seller is to educate yourself on every aspect of buying a home, and listen to your intuition.

If you decide to go with an agent, your best bet is to interview agents until you find one with whom you are comfortable. Do not sign anything until you feel you have found the right one, and be careful about signing buyers' agreements, as some of them may ask that you promise things you can't deliver (promising that you won't bail out on the agent if you find a good For Sale by Owner property, for example).

Make sure your agent has time for you and is interested in helping you. Recommendations from friends and family are always good, because if a smart agent gets business from more than one person in a family, she knows she has good customers for life, and will do a great job to keep them happy.

It's More Than a Roof Over Your Head—It's an Investment
A home is not only a place to hang your hat. It is also probably the biggest investment you will ever make. If the home you are looking at is not a good investment, you are better off not buying it.

Here are a few things to consider when buying a home:

1. In order for an investment to be worth your money, you have to be able to sell it quickly for what it's worth. If you buy a home knowing that you are stuck there for the rest of your life, or that you'll never afford to fix the things that are wrong with it, you have made an unwise investment.
2. Is the neighborhood safe? If not, it will be hard to sell your home when the time comes, regardless of its charms.
3. Are property values in that area going up? If property values in your area are not climbing or staying steady, you will lose money from your investment.
4. Never, ever buy a house that has a "non-disclosure" clause. This means that the seller does not have to tell you about certain things that have happened in the house. Maybe it was used as a meth lab and harbors toxic chemicals, maybe it was used as a brothel and you can expect strange people to come to your door looking for sex or drugs, maybe people were murdered there and there is some bad energy hanging around, and maybe it's got a bad foundation issue and it's

about to fall down. Regardless, a non-disclosure clause shows that there is something to hide that will affect a person's desire to buy that home.
5. If you are interested in living in an environmentally clean and sustainable community, research intentional housing communities, co-housing options, and Eco-Villages. Sometimes you can acquire a wonderful place to live with other like-minded home owners and can exchange services such as gardening, child care, animal care, etc. with trusted neighbors. Such communities are rare at this time, but are becoming more common all the time.
6. A Home Inspection Report is normally required by your mortgage company. If not, get one anyway. Sometimes the seller will be willing to pay for and perform some (if not all) necessary repairs, or they will have to make those repairs in order for the home to be financed. Additionally, you might discover something that makes you not want that place after all, and you can almost always walk away from the deal without losing any money if the repairs that need to be made are too extensive for the buyer or seller to perform under the current contract.
7. If you are looking at a condo, make sure to ask what things are covered in your condo dues, as you will sometimes have to pay for things out of your own pocket. For example, some condos require that you do your own snow removal, and that if you don't they will fine you.
8. Also, if you are buying a condo, make sure all common areas are clean and well cared for. If there is a bunch of junk in the common areas, you don't want to live there. If the roof of the carport is sagging, you don't want to live there. Pay attention to these things, as they affect your property value and show the quality of your neighbors.
9. If your condo project has a parking space for you and you live in a city and don't have a car, you may be able to rent your parking space out!
10. Did you know that a portion of the interest you pay on your house can be written off your taxes? This is one reason why sometimes it's cheaper to own than to rent.
11. Do research to know what things mean. Did you know that if a house has a septic system, you won't be able to flush your tampons, that you shouldn't use bleach, and that you will have to use your garbage disposal sparingly? Did you know that if there is an electrical easement on you property, the electric company has the right to rip up that portion of your yard if they need access to their equipment? Don't let anything go over your head. If you hear a word you don't understand, ask (and make sure you understand) what it means.

♦ ♦ ♦

Having a great place to live is one of life's pleasures. You and your child deserve to live in an environment that is safe, stimulating, comforting, efficient, and helps you to reach your life goals. By now you know that there are certain things in life you can't control, but your environment is not one of them. Whether you live by yourself in a tiny one bedroom apartment, a bedroom in your mom's house, a mansion with several roommates; whether you have a houseful of antiques or a couple of plants and an air mattress on the floor; whether you own, rent, or live rent-free with family, make your home a place that you are happy to be in and happy to come home to. A lot of your work in the next three years will be done in your home. Make sure your home is deserving of your time, your dreams, and your presence.

Chapter Ten

Work/Life Balance

If you happen to be one of the few single pregnant women whose parents are taking care of you, or who is otherwise in a situation that doesn't require you to work, that is fabulous. If this is the case, it is extremely important that you use this time to advance yourself and program yourself for success in life because it might be a long time, if ever, that you get another extended block of time off from some kind of work. Please read this chapter in its entirety, as it contains important information about things you will do as a single parent when you return to the workforce, and will help you develop an understanding of the sociological setting of the workplace: how it relates to women, mothers, and single mothers—and how you can ensure that anyone's potential judgments about your situation won't stop you from getting what you need and deserve.

Before we discuss your work situation, we will discuss something even more important: Your life. After all, you may not always have your job, but you will always have your life. Pregnancy and early parenthood—especially when single—can turn a person into a shut-in. But even the biggest introvert needs to understand that opportunities don't often come knocking at your door. Little social miracles happen every day: You go out to get a cup of decaf in the morning, strike up a conversation with the barista, and learn that her sister has an opening for an infant at her day care, which is conveniently located near your house. Or you find a posting for that perfect job at the grocery store bulletin board, or you drop your friend off at home to find that her husband's best friend is just your type. Miracles *do* happen—don't forget this, even if it seems you have been due for a long time. But the truth is this: They often can't find you if you're not looking for them, and the more people you interact with in a day, the greater your chances for being noticed by the right person for the right reason for that right blessing.

At the beginning of a pregnancy, you may hear many women say things like "Life, as I know it, is over." It is certain that there will be changes, especially if you're college-aged and it seems that all anyone ever does is go out to bars or rock and roll concerts. Yes, your days of hanging out at the local watering hole are a thing of the past for a while, and certain fun activities that leave you standing or waiting in restroom lines for any length of time will quickly become not-so-fun; but you will soon learn that spending money in pubs was never really where the real fun was anyway, and you can always get back to anything your pregnancy made you miss. Sure, some pessimists will still say that life is over, but I say that your real and meaningful life is just beginning, and this book is your first step towards making *life* work for *you*. There is a lot of fun to be had in this world, and pregnancy will not prevent you from being let in on the action. Read this chapter for some ideas on how to fill your time with productive fun and frolic, and for some ideas on how you can simplify your life for more time, money, and pleasure.

Doing and Being
What is it that you've always wanted to do, but something has been stopping you? Maybe you've always wanted to learn to paint, to dance, speak another language, or play a musical instrument, but someone told you that you weren't talented, you weren't smart, or you weren't coordinated enough, and you believed them?

An inspiring story from my own neighborhood: A friend's son's father, who happens to be obese, had repeatedly told the son that he was destined to be obese as well. "That's how we are built," he would say. "You might as well accept who you are and learn to be happy despite it."

While I'm all for people being happy, to be obese was not this child's choice, nor was it his physiological sentence—it was his programming. He was told by his own father that there was nothing he could do to change his physical and social struggle that was apparent to anyone who would observe him slowly walking to the bus stop alone and using all of his focus to avoid icy patches on the sidewalk. While I'm not sure what happened to this child to break him free of this programming, he can now be seen jogging through the neighborhood daily. He is extremely healthy, and is capable of physical feats far beyond what most people can achieve. To observe him now, one would never know of his former sentence. This transition into a physically fit man happened in his last two years of high school, just in time for adulthood.

My sister, another example, was never an athlete. Between the two of us, she was the smart and bookish one (I was the athlete and the clown). Three years ago she started doing yoga two or three times a week. At the time of this writing she is 48 years old, and has done her first ever back bend from a standing position.

Do you have any similar programming? While I would agree that some people have more talent and ability than others, and it is easier to excel at certain goals—playing the violin, for example—when a person starts in their youth. But most people can achieve a satisfying level of success at anything they set their mind to if they just get over the idea that life is a race or a competition. True, you will sometimes encounter someone who seems to relish the idea that they are more talented than you are, but don't let this person dictate how you measure your level of success. Also, you may find after years of dance class that you just don't have the right stuff to be a performer—but if that's the case, who cares? You got three years of exercise figuring that out. Measure your success based on how you have improved at anything since you started. Furthermore, assuming that you are pregnant, you are still young, so it's not time to tell yourself that you could never do what you want to do. A fiddler in a well-liked Irish folk band in my town didn't start fiddling until he was fifty. While there may be a reader or two who happens to be in their forties, the high likelihood is that you are much younger than that, so you cannot fall back on your age as a reason for not trying to do what you want to do. Finally, from what I've seen, it's hard to believe that you would be one of the people who just can't do *anything* well. Such people are extremely rare, and I hold the belief that their inability is at least partially programming, and that they come with their own special set of unrecognized or uncovered gifts.

That said, what do you dream about being able to do? Once you start something, bear in mind that it's perfectly fine to abandon it after a while if you have found that you simply don't enjoy the activity. But never give up on something because you haven't mastered it overnight. You have your whole life ahead of you, and life is not a race.

Furthermore, what you do for fun does not have to be something other people appreciate. Doing something you enjoy that is not particularly productive is your right. If window shopping makes you feel alive, do it. If internet gaming makes you feel like you rule the world, do it. If binge watching an entire TV series gets your creative juices flowing, kick back with some popcorn and live like you want. The important thing here is to enjoy your life on your own terms and love your inner child because you are her advocate.

Let's take a look at a few things you can do, productive or not, to add some spice to your life. We will start by how you can enhance your life by getting out, staying in, keeping your job and career on track, and then making sure you can blend it all together to make life both manageable and fun.

Getting Out
Classes and Workshops
No matter what you want to do, there is a person out there who can teach you how to do it: yoga, hula hooping, basket weaving, jewelry making, dancing, playing an instrument, bonsai, pottery, cooking, etc. Sometimes you can even find free demonstrations sponsored by a food company, at a faire of some kind, a book store, or a church. At this time, I wouldn't recommend committing to anything long-term, as you can't be sure you will be able to keep the commitment, but short-term classes (maybe four weeks) or one-night workshops can provide enough exposure to help you decide if you want to continue, and

you always leave a workshop knowing *something* new. And while some things require you to continue to take classes to develop and grow, there are other things that only require you to expose yourself to the basics, at which time you can continue your education through videos or fining a community. If you try something and decide it's not for you, at least you will have learned what you *don't* want to do, and this is just as much a part of life as learning what you *do* want to do, right?

The only kind of classes that wouldn't be recommended are those which expose you to toxic chemicals or are too physically strenuous or dangerous (maybe not the time to try sky diving). Working with stained glass, or working with film photo chemicals, etc., is something you may want to put off until it's safer.

Finding a Likeminded Tribe

Some interests might not require you to take classes. And sometimes you have taken enough classes to know what you're doing, but you'd like other people to do it with. Improving your Spanish speaking skills, for example, might best be achieved by getting together with other Spanish speakers, and sometimes it's safest to go hiking with a group of people rather than alone. You may want to find other people who are interested in natural parenting, dancing, political activism, hunting or fishing, bartering and trading, carpooling, working out, spirituality and meditation, gardening, etc.

The first step to finding these people would be to register on a site such as meetup.com, and browsing the different groups that you might be interested in joining. In my experience, registering for a meet-up group can take a person's social life from being dull and boring to being filled to the gills. You may even decide to form your own meet-up for single pregnant women.

Meals out

No, you don't have to break the bank just to have a nice meal out on the town, and one of the great things about being in your second or third trimester is that everything tastes delicious! Sushi bars are great places to have inexpensive and healthy meals (avoid anything raw while you are pregnant, and be aware of the types of fish that have high mercury content), Mexican restaurants normally serve complimentary chips and salsa and boast a fun, social atmosphere, and becoming a regular at your local breakfast place is a great way to meet your neighbors (no, you don't need company—bring a newspaper, homework, book, laptop, or journal to keep you company in the event that nobody strikes up a conversation with you). Any place that has a bar to sit at is usually a good place to eat, read the paper, socialize, and just be out of the house.

After a few consistent appearances at the same place and possibly the same time, the staff may start to notice your regularity. They begin to know your order, know your name, know your habits… this might not seem too exciting, but it easier for miracles to find you when you've demonstrated your dependability to the universe. For example, once in a blue moon people will notice that there's also a nice looking gentleman who regularly sits at your habitual table two hours after you've left, and sometimes these people decide that you should meet. Or, after shopping for a dresser all over town, you strike up a conversation with your server and find that she is selling a beautiful antique dresser for a price you can afford!

Going out to eat *every day* would be a costly habit, but you may be able to eat out at a breakfast place, a sushi place, a sandwich shop, or a Mexican restaurant once a week. Just make sure to choose meals that don't cost more than if you'd made them at home.

Sports and Outdoor Activities
True, there are many things that you won't be able to do (snowboarding, horseback riding…), and many more that you won't even want to do (I was surprised to find that even badminton can be painful and awkward when you're pregnant). But depending on how athletic you are and how far along you are in your pregnancy, this might be a great time to do some mellow outdoor activities that are not too strenuous on your body to get you connected to your world. I learned to sea kayak in my second trimester, and was up in the mountains picking berries (although not very quickly) into my eighth month.

Although some of you may have special circumstances that prevent you from doing physical things, most pregnant women can swim, walk, take mellow short-distance bike rides, garden (even window gardening can soothe your soul), pick berries, shop, play croquet, dance, camp, and fish practically until they're ready to give birth. A good rule is to make sure that you can take a sit-down break no matter what you're doing, and bring along plenty of water, snacks, cab fare, cellphone, sunscreen, and a safe DEET-free and preferably natural mosquito repellent.

Support Groups and Spiritual Communities
If you live in an urban area, you can find support groups and spiritual communities for practically any situation or interest. If you don't live in an urban area, you may still have access to these communities. Check Craigslist or Meetup.com to see if there is a support community that's right for you.

Staying In
Depending on your energy level and mobility, going out may be more trouble than it's worth, but that doesn't mean you need to be lonely or bored. There are lots of ways to make sure the party finds you at home.

House Parties

There are as many reasons to party as there are people on this earth. You can have your friends over to knit, to watch movies, to play games, to sunbathe, to write, to discuss books, to go for a walk; and just the other day I was invited to a scrap-booking party with some local ladies just because I came into their store.

Remember to always have a variety of snacks and drinks available for your guests so nobody has to leave early on account of simply being hungry or thirsty. Always consider the needs of the dieters, the diabetics, the teetotalers, the vegetarians and vegans, the people with food allergies, and even try to accommodate the smokers by putting an ashtray on the deck if you can (just because they smoke doesn't mean they're not your friends). If you're having trouble thinking of what to make, you can never go wrong with a vegetable plate and dip, chips and salsa, and cheese and crackers. For drinks, have some water, juice, and maybe hot tea, beer, and wine, depending on your guests.

On a more cautious note, pay attention to your guest list. Don't invite two people who dislike each other, and if you think certain friends may get too drunk and rowdy or disrespect your home, it's time to find some new friends. At this time in your life, you need to surround yourself with only positive influences.

Game Night

You can start a great tradition by hosting a monthly game night with your friends. This is a good way to keep in touch with what's going on and laugh heartily. Scrabble, Monopoly, and various card games are great for traditionalists, and there are some newer favorites to choose from as well. Take a friend to the toy store and browse the aisles for what looks like fun. Again, if you're hosting, remember the snacks. Nothing falls flat more quickly than a party with starving guests.

Recycling Parties

We've all heard the mantra: Reduce, reuse, recycle. And budget-minded and eco-minded people are wise to regard this as a permanent change in our culture rather than a trend.

Every December 26th I have a "Boxing Day" party, in which I invite all my friends over. The highlight of this party is the gift exchange: people bring a gift they received that they cannot personally use: A shirt that doesn't fit, an item the recipient already has, or something that's just plain not their style. As one who has sensitive skin, I can't use most scented skin products. Last year at my party, my guests were fighting over a set of scented bath oils I had received from a co-worker. I was happy to know that the scented oils were wanted by someone, and had found a good home.

You can also have a clothing swap. Have all your friends bring over clothes they no longer want, and let everyone trade or just take the clothes they want. As the hostess, you might arrange to take what's left over to the Salvation Army, get a receipt, and write the donation off your taxes, or if there's anything really great, maybe you can even take them to the consignment shop and earn some more money!

You can plan a recycling party for practically any reason. Be creative, and have a great time!

Dinners at Home

Everybody's got to eat. Might as well make a social event out of it, right? Task one of your friends or family members with bringing a beverage, salad, or side dish. If you have never considered yourself much of a cook, now is time for you to start making tasty, healthy meals to impress your little one, your friends, maybe your future partner, and most importantly, yourself. Sure, you can learn from a cookbook, but it's also fun to take a class from a local co-op or grocery chain. If you don't have the right gear to cook what you want, you can *always* find cheap kitchen stuff at garage sales or second-hand stores (remember to wash everything thoroughly and make sure you have all the parts to anything you buy). Familiarize yourself with local traditional foods using those food items that are fresh and readily available in your area, and branch out to the exciting and exotic after you have a handle on what's growing outside your back door.

Fun on the Internet

Gaming:

Yes, I'm sure you've heard all the rumors: you've heard that interactive on-line gaming will turn you into a nerd, a spinster, and will ultimately steal your soul. But I am here to tell you the truth: If you're a creative, intelligent, computer-savvy and fantasy-oriented person, interactive on-line gaming can be a lot of fun, and can connect you with local and international people who have similar interests. I even know two women who met their (high quality) husbands playing an online role playing games. One came all the way from Denmark to Alaska to meet his future wife, the other from Sweden. Yup—it happens.

For three years I spent about two nights a week living as a monk fighting villains and dragons in a game called Everquest. I made friends all over the world, many of whom I still talk to, many of them single parents, pregnant women, or people whose physical limitations prevented them from having an active social life outside the home. During those three years I never had to worry about driving in dangerous conditions, cab fare after a night of drinking, or paying a babysitter in order to interact with people and have a good time. I looked forward to the next time I could log on and see my friends in our fantasy world, and I didn't feel like I was missing out on life simply because I was a single mother. Yes, I did enjoy my Internet gaming and played often, but never considered myself an addict—all my responsibilities were taken care of, all my bills were paid, and I would always warn my friends that I might have to leave the game quickly if my baby started to cry.

When computer updates became too costly and high maintenance, when my son got a little older, and when I started to acquire more opportunities and obligations outside my home, I started to lose interest in my game, and eventually stopped playing. However, I wouldn't give back my Everquest experience for the world, as it helped me get through what may have been a more difficult time without it.

If you enjoy on-line Internet gaming, simply make sure your life does not get out of balance. Pay your bills, be sure to exercise and spend some time outside, take care of your child's needs, and have a guilt-free great time!

Internet Dating
Okay, sure: Now might not be the right time. But when the time is right, you may learn that the Internet is just about the only place left to meet men when your life is extremely busy. We are often warned that we can find some pretty shady characters on the Internet, but can't the same be said for the physical world? One thing that's really great about the Internet is that you can often find people who are at least somewhat pre-screened to echo your own values. Take for example Vegetarian singles sites, Green Singles, Equestrian Singles, eHarmony, and of course Match.com... I even heard of one dating site for people who are *either* rich or good-looking (but I haven't visited yet, ha ha). Before you try your hand at Internet dating, though, make a list of those qualities you want in a partner *as well as* those you will not accept: Don't ignore a person's values, behavior, political alignment, or lifestyle, as these are all potential deal-breakers. Don't have extremely high expectations (sometimes a man will look great until you dig deeper), and never lower your standards (if he says *anything* that makes you flinch, cut it off right then and there before you get attached: He's just a picture on the computer screen until you meet him, and pictures are illusions). Make sure dates are in public and have a time limit the first few times, and don't give you your phone number until you are sure this person has the appropriate boundaries not to text you at midnight or demand attention when it's not in your best interest to give it.

My own Internet dating experience has been a mixed bag. I have met some men with whom I had long-term relationships or general friendships and relationships of mutual respect. I've also met a few toads. Remember that while there are good people out there, there are more people you have to be careful of. You don't owe anyone anything, but you owe it to yourself to screen people thoroughly, listen to your intuition, refuse to give out your number until you're ready, and bail on any situation that makes you itch.

If you do meet a string of men who simply don't have the right stuff, or you seem to be attracting the same unacceptable type over and over (cheap, superficial, angry, dishonest, etc.), take a step back—maybe hide your profile or just don't check messages for a while and consider analyzing and refining your profile narrative or photos. Sometimes the energy of putting yourself out there can be painful or toxic, but sometimes it's fun. Just listen to yourself about whether Internet dating is good or bad for you at any time.

Workin' It
By now you probably well know that while some people think of a single woman continuing an unsupported pregnancy as a hero, a great many people think otherwise. Having been single throughout my son's entire youth, I am always surprised when single-mothers-as-the-result-of-divorce will broadcast their status as single mothers whenever they suffer any sort of perceived injustice, believing that to do so might earn them sympathy, understanding, or special, preferential treatment. The truth is that it usually does just the opposite. When it comes to your job, your status as a single mother-to-be should be, at best, an afterthought—and this should continue to be the case after you are a mother, whether single or partnered.

In the workplace, it is important that you portray yourself as neither a hero nor a martyr. Instead, portray yourself as a worker with the same limits and capabilities as anyone else—nothing more, nothing less. While we all know that your challenges likely are and will be far greater than those of the majority of your peers, you have made a life choice to continue your pregnancy and be a mother to your child. If others in the workplace end up suffering because of your choice, you are likely to alienate your team members and disappoint your supervisors, and will certainly be viewed as one who is not contributing appropriately, which affects your job stability.

Furthermore, sometimes you learn long after-the-fact that this person over here was going through a divorce, that person was caring for his mother who had cancer (which was the secret of his enviable weight loss), or you learn at the holiday party that this woman is the single mother of a downs syndrome child. Why didn't you know any of this stuff? It's because when someone values their job, they leave their baggage at home. Yes, your circumstances are challenging, and so are theirs. Sadly, pregnancy in the workplace can place a target right on your back, and being single makes it even bigger.

If you are (or will be) in management, you may one day have to take someone aside and tell them that they can no longer discuss their breakup while at work. You may have to tell a new mother that she needs to limit her parenting/ day care/grandma/Halloween costume logistics calls in common workspace and that all such calls have to be completed during her lunch hour or 15-minute breaks. You may have to tell someone that if they are late one more time, they will lose their job. My goal is to ensure that you are not the one who needs to be told these things.

Regardless, there are things that need to be done right away. If the company you work for has more than 50 employees in the city or county (municipality, borough) where you work, you need to get into contact with your HR department and apply for FMLA, which is family medical leave. This protects your job in the event that you have (or an immediate family member has) medical issues that prevent you from being in attendance at work for a period of time. Depending on your company, you will likely have to take all of your paid leave before the FMLA benefits kick in. If your pregnancy or parenthood causes you to be out of the office for a time that exceeds your FMLA benefit, you may be able to claim short-term disability—which isn't much, but it's something.

You will have to tell your supervisor about your pregnancy so they are not blindsided when they receive the FMLA paperwork. Let your boss know that you don't anticipate taking any time off unnecessarily and that it's important to you that you continue to do a good job and are perceived as a contributor in the workplace, but that you never know what's going to happen down the road so you are being proactive in protecting yourself and the company. Let your boss know that while you realize the pregnancy will eventually be common knowledge, you are not going to bring any attention to it. Tell her you will endeavor to schedule all your medical appointments at times that you are not working, but if absences are necessary, ask if there are preferred days and times to schedule appointments, or days that you absolutely can't be absent, how much notice is needed for a medical appointment, etc. Any decent boss will appreciate your conscientiousness, and might just assure you that you are safe to do what needs to be done to keep yourself healthy through this time.

Beyond your chat with your supervisor, following are some rules to live by to ensure things are smooth at work.

#1: At work, silence is your friend. I'm not a big fan of hiding, and I think people need to live out loud in their personal lives. But your work life is *not* your personal life. I recommend avoiding the topic of your pregnancy with your co-workers as long as you can, other than with those who are your true and personal friends. Don't freak out, however, if people suspect or learn about your pregnancy without you telling them. It will be common knowledge soon enough. Just don't bring unnecessary attention to it. If people ask for details about your situation, say as little as possible without seeming itchy about it. The less intriguing you make your personal business, the less interested people will be. If a pregnant co-worker has been suffering with extreme morning sickness and you have not, and she happens to broach a conversation with you, give her suggestions for how to deal with it rather than coming out and saying you haven't experienced that symptom. If you have worked out with your boss that you are going to take all twelve weeks of your FMLA and then go on short-term disability until you're ready to come back to work (which can sometimes happen when you are a good worker who is appreciated by their boss), keep that between you and her/him. If your baby's father is on a rampage and might come in to your place at work, calmly notify your HR department (or your supervisor) that there have been threats and to please document any misbehavior so you can involve the authorities in forcing him to stop. If people ask why he is reacting so, wave it away and say, "His anger is so illogical it's not even worth trying to explain. His behavior will be stopped. Lesson learned: he's nuts. Moving on." Let the drama be *his*, not yours.

If you have medical issues—or your child has medical issues in the future—it's best if you don't give details unless they take up fewer than thirty seconds of your boss's or co-worker's time and doesn't force them to think about *your* problems. Consider the difference between these phrases: #1: "I have learned that my child is allergic to several things, and there's a huge learning curve in knowing how to manage it all, so it's taking up a bit of my energy." #2: "I learned that my son is allergic to peanuts, eggs and corn! Oh my god, those things are in everything. There's almost nothing that he can eat. I will have to read labels for the rest of my life, and he is going to have to carry an epi-pen! And corn: Did you know that even some cellophane wrappers of prescriptions have corn in them, and so it contaminates the very medicine the child needs for the allergy in the first place? Halloween is never going to be fun. I'm going to be on pins and needles worrying for the rest of my life."

Everyone has challenges. People will be sympathetic enough when they know a situation is serious. It's not necessary to ensure they understand all that you are going through, and not recommended to pull on a person's energy in order to ensure they completely understand, especially at work.

#2: Keep your baggage at home. Again, advise your supervisor if there is a chance that you will have to take an unscheduled personal call regarding your medical issues, legal issues, or your child. This will help communicate to her that you respect the company's time and that you acknowledge that this is a special circumstance, not the way it will always be. If you need any special accommodation—a bigger chair, or to do a certain task that keeps you away from the public because there is a chance that you're going to get sick—communicate that quietly to your supervisor, and always thank her and let her know that will help you to focus and be productive. If you had a hard time getting out of bed this morning or you were up all night thinking of how you were going to respond to your baby father's rude email, keep that to yourself. Sure, you may broadcast in the lunch room that you need a referral for a good family law attorney, but if people ask why, you can just answer "custody, child support. You know…" And if a friend's recommendation does not work out, they don't need to know the details why.

Practice the poker face: Again, people will say stupid things. People will say insensitive things. People will ask questions about things that are none of their business. While the people who do this don't always have malicious intentions, most mature people will respect your privacy. If someone hurts you with their words or questions, don't let them know you're hurt. Again, if their intentions are to make you feel bad, it's not interesting to see you doing well. If people at work do say hurtful, nosy, or inappropriate things, there are a couple of ways you can deal with this. #1: Pretend you don't know what they're talking about. Look at them like they just said something in a language you don't understand at all. If they press, turn it around on them: Look them square in the eye without looking upset at all, and ask, "Why would you ask such a question/ say such a thing?" Or: "I know you didn't *mean* to say that, but…" Hold their gaze until the look away, and then walk away as though it neve happened. This should either shut them up, or force them to expose themselves as a nosy bitch. #2: Smile smugly like you have a secret, shrug, and walk away. #3: Give them nothing. No reaction at all. If it continues, talk to your supervisor about it. Calmly say, "I have chosen not to discuss the details of my personal situation at work, and it seems so-and-so is getting frustrated with my not spilling the details to her. I am not sure there's anything that should be done about it—I just wanted to advise you." She will probably ask you to document what was said and when, as well as any future occurrences.

Simplify Your Life for More Time, Money, and Pleasure

While I was pregnant and for a few years after my son was born, I went through a financially very hard time, and the financial hardships I had experienced repeated when both of my parents had long-term medical emergencies that required me to quit my job in order to take care of them. During those times, I had to make some serious lifestyle adjustments in order to stay afloat—but in those years following my pregnancy and before my family emergency, I found myself living a lifestyle that was more sustainable, less expensive, healthier, and ultimately more pleasurable that the lifestyle I'd had before. (It should be noted that having to take care of my parents was much harder than my pregnancy and parenthood experience—but thankfully, the financial part of my struggle was something I had experienced and knew how to handle. I knew what needed to be done, so I got through it. The habits that I formed during my pregnancy and early parenthood have stayed with me through times that they were no longer necessary for survival. I don't intend to laud these things over anyone else, as it might truly make you happier to have a new car than to have one that's paid off. It might be more practical for you to pay full price for an item so you can return it rather than take the time to find it on eBay and sell it if it doesn't work out. Going out to a movie and getting the expensive concessions might truly lift your spirits in a way that nothing else can—and this book is about making *you* happy and fulfilled, not turning you into a clone. My intention is strictly to provide strategies you may have never considered, based on how you were raised and your social circle. And although making major life adjustments is not within everyone's abilities, sometimes if we have time to do what needs to be done, life can be far less expensive than we have grown to expect.

Before we go into potential sustainability issues, let's consider what natural parenting experts consider to be decisions that positively impact the baby: Breastfeeding, co-sleeping (sleeping with the baby), and staying at home (or otherwise with the baby) for as long as possible before returning to work or otherwise separating your from your baby. There's even a group called NINO (nine in nine out) that touts the benefits of "wearing" your baby for at least nine months in order to help the child grow to be secure and stable and have a good relationship with his or her mother. We are starting to learn that the old-fashioned practice of consistently letting a baby "cry it out" or forcing a baby to sleep away from its mother can actually create harmful emotional detachment issues that last well into adulthood.

It is also recommended to limit or completely banish chemicals in cleaning products, gardening products, and food (yours *and* the baby's).

Despite our knowing what's believed to be best for the baby, sometimes our reality dictates that we must cut corners in one area or another in order to meet our needs, which is one of the reasons I refrain from judging any pregnancy, birthing, or parenting decision that my reader decides to make. The unfortunate fact is that our culture does not bend to the needs of parents, let alone single parents! But sometimes a new mother can successfully limit her financial needs enough to make choices that will deliver long-term benefits for her and her baby. Although you are entitled to have your own values and comfort level, the following are some suggestions that might help give you enough wiggle room to more freely decide what your priorities are.

Break the daily mocha/latte/espresso habit. If you make coffee at home, you will save approximately three dollars a day—that's $90.00 a month! If you are too addicted to coffee shop lattes, bring your own cup, and depending on your chosen coffee place, you can save money every day—but you can save much more by mastering how to make the perfect up at home and bringing it with you in a travel mug.

Save coupons for products you use and sign up for your supermarket's "customer loyalty" or "rewards" savings cards. One of my local supermarkets sends me $15.00 worth of coupons every month. Another not only rewards me with savings on products I buy, but also gives me air miles and gas discounts. Sometimes the register computers generate coupons for products I have bought in the past. Based on all these factors, I save about least $30.00 a month. I carry a small pouch in my purse to store coupons I have a chance of using, and I can check my special custom discounts in real time on the store's app on my smartphone.

Bring your own shopping bags to the market. Yes, in some places this is becoming mandatory. If not, some stores offer a $.05 refund on your grocery bill for ever bag you provide. It's good for the Earth, and good for your pocketbook.

Shop at your local farmers' markets. Fruits and veggies are sometimes cheaper when you buy direct from the farmer, and are better for your local economy. Sometimes farmers will throw in extra items for free.

Buy in bulk when products you use are on sale. Bulk shopping is not always practical, and a good deal can sometimes tempt you into buying something you don't need. But if you use a product and are sure it won't spoil before you use it all (always check expiration dates, as that might be the reason they're on sale), take advantage of bulk savings opportunities.

Bring a sack lunch with you when eating out is a convenience rather than an occasion. Eating out is fun, but should be on your own terms, and should only be done when you are truly interested in the food you're eating, the company you're keeping, or the ambiance of where you'll be eating. If your habit of eating out consists of a rushed one-hour meal on for lunch at whatever restaurant is nearby, bring your lunch to work instead, and only eat out when you can truly relax and enjoy your meal or make it a social event. Of course, don't force yourself to stay inside if you really enjoy leaving the office for your lunch break, but depending on your job, you may be able to work through your lunch and get off an hour earlier. If there is a fridge at your work, get into the habit of stocking the fridge and freezer so that you can either choose to accept an interesting lunch invitation or eat the food you have when you don't want to leave the office.

Make second-hand shopping a habit. Many years ago, I challenged myself not to purchase any truly new clothes other than socks, underwear, shoes (if needed) and possibly swimsuits, for the entire year. Guess what? I still looked good. These days, the price of a new pair of the latest designer jeans no longer makes me cry—it makes me laugh. Why would I buy a $200.00 pair of jeans when I can get the same jeans for $75.00—better yet, if I can find a comparable pair at American Eagle for half that? If I am interested in a popular item that I can get for a deep discount second-hand (my last experiment was a robotic vacuum), I search for it online. *Lots* of people buy things and then wait to learn how to use it until after it can no longer be returned, and then learn it doesn't suit their needs, or they are moving and don't want to take it with, etc. Getting things like books and CDs used is a no-brainer. Now that this is a habit, I wouldn't shop any other way.

Buy your seasonal clothes and gear on sale the year before you need them. If your boots, winter coats, or swimsuits will be worn out at the end of the season, make sure to hit the end-of-the season sales that year—you could save yourself hundreds of dollars, and you won't have to scramble to find a good winter coat after the temperatures have dropped. *But for now*, be careful with anticipating your future size until a year after your baby is born.

Stop using expensive (and potentially harmful) chemical cleaners. You can clean just about anything in your home with vinegar, baking soda, hydrogen peroxide, and tea tree (Melaleuca) oil, all of which can be purchased in bulk at superstores like Costco. Look on the internet to find out how these products can be used to keep your home clean.

If you anticipate that you have some jobs that are too tough to be handled by these natural products, my mother once told me that the only cleaner a person needs is Bon Ami scouring powder, which costs about a dollar a can, and can last as long as a year or longer, depending on how big your house is and how quickly you clean up messes.

If there are products you use that make life easier on you, by all means use them (I'm a big fan of the Mister Clean Magic Eraser, and my sister loves the smell of Mrs. Meyer's Clean Day products). But don't believe you have to have a specific cleaner for the toilet, and a different one for the stove, and yet another one for the bathtub when it can all be done just as quickly and just as well with a scouring powder.

You don't need a price club membership. Instead, go with a friend or relative who has a membership, and calculate what you owe afterwards. I go on Costco "dates" about three times a year, and I bring along a list of what I need. I save money on the membership, and I'm less tempted to buy things I don't need than if I were to have constant access to the entire warehouse.

Keep an eye on your utilities. At the time of this writing, natural gas in my area is expensive. But I have cut my gas bill way down by getting an electric water kettle and a toaster oven, and using space heaters in the colder spots in my house. In the winter, my son and I sleep with hot water bottles rather than turning the heat up all night. Also, anything in your house with a digital clock or a light on is sucking electricity. Turn everything off when it's not in use. I put my TV, Roku box, etc., on a power strip so I don't have to cut the power on multiple items when I'm done watching TV, as does my son with his video game set-up.

Can you save money on your garbage bill? Some towns and cities offer recycling incentives by charging you based on the weight of your garbage. Try to limit the amount of waste you produce by recycling, plan your meals in order to use up all of your perishables, and if you live in a rural area, it is easy to compost your food scraps.

If you have a dog and are in the habit of cooking with only natural ingredients, certain dogs can sometimes eat your leftovers if they don't contain grapes, bread, onions, garlic, chocolate, unnatural amounts of sodium and sugar, and fried foods—but the ability to do this varies widely from dog to dog. My last dog could eat anything at all, but my current dog gets gassy if she eats anything but her regular dry dog food. Please do your own research before feeding your dog too many people foods, and mix small parts of people food with larger amounts of their regular food to help protect them from an upset stomach.

Don't throw away the dark meat! If you're like most people, you will buy and cook a rotisserie chicken, take off the convenient and accessible meat, and then throw the carcass away. If you're industrious, you will boil the carcass to soften the "harder to get" meat, remove it from the bones, freeze it if you don't have an immediate use for it, use it to make tacos, chicken soup, casserole, or dog food, and use the boiled (chicken stock) water to make soup or to use in another recipe that calls for chicken stock (a 16oz can or box of organic chicken stock costs about four dollars). If you do this, you can pour the cooled down chicken stock into clean plastic yogurt or sour cream containers and freeze them. Always make sure to put the date on the containers and revolve your supply.

Have meals *with* your baby. After your baby starts eating, it is a good idea to have a few jars of (hopefully organic) baby food at home, but it will save you time, money, and will be better for your baby if you can make your own baby foods out of items you will be using for your own meals. Avocados are good for the baby and are good for keeping *your* skin looking young, so smash up some avocado for the baby. Bananas are considered nature's perfect food. Look at the ingredients of the baby food that's in jars: peas, squash, potatoes… mash them up yourself (but do so before you add any salt). As your baby gets more tolerant of food, get a baby food grinder (or a bullet-style blender) and grind up a bit of whatever you're eating (watch out for popular allergens though, and avoid salt, sugar, and use spices sparingly). There's little reason to buy baby food if what you're eating is healthy enough!

Use up what you already have. If the shampoo you have is not your favorite brand but still works well enough, use it up before you buy any more. If your bathroom cabinets are full of half-used bottles of everything and you know you aren't going to use them, see if you can unload them on a friend for a *great* deal (keep in mind that a *great* deal is $.50 for a half-used $7.00 bottle of shampoo. Don't try to get maximum dollar value for used products. Used bath and body products and makeup cannot be sold on E-bay or Craigslist.org due to hygiene issues, so appreciate any money your get for something you will not use). Another thing you can do is donate these items to a homeless shelter or abused women's home. Call up and find out if they accept such items, save your receipt, and write the donation off your taxes.

Walk, bike, carpool, or use public transportation when feasible. Walking and biking are not only good for the environment, but for *you* too! Carpooling can save you tons of money, and public transportation can save you money, get you to where you're going, and give you time to read a book (or bond with your baby) when otherwise you'd be staring at the road. Many Americans have a strong affinity for their cars, but whether or not a car is truly an asset to you depends on many factors. I have some adult friends in Europe and San Francisco who have never even gotten their driver's license because public transportation addresses their needs to get anywhere they need to go.

If you are lucky/industrious enough to live nearby your work and day care, walking or biking gives you the added benefit of exercising every day without having to schedule it. This can do wonders for your overall physical and mental health as well as your pocketbook.

If you have a long commute to work, you can sometimes find a carpool through craigslist, and sometimes your city's public transportation has carpooling options. In my city, if you (or they) can find enough people, the city provides the carpool group with a van. Each member of the carpool pays a certain amount of money, and one person is the steward of the van. The responsibility of the steward is to keep the van clean and pick everyone up on time in the morning. Sometimes the steward pays less than everyone else, and sometimes pays nothing at all. Depending on the resources available in your area combined with your punctuality, driving record, and dependability, this might be something for you to consider.

Don't over-invest in unproductive "ass time." It's amazing to learn how many people have perceived cable TV as a necessity—but it seems that the people have spoken and times they are-a-changing: Nobody wants to have 101 channels of crap available to them just because they want to watch their favorite show on a cable channel. People are now opting for having streaming TV, or Roku box or some other streaming device, and being able to cherry-pick the channels and shows they want. If you have wireless internet, this option is very cost-effective. If streaming TV shows is still too expensive for you or is not a priority, rabbit ears still work. ABC, NBC, PBS, and CBS are available without any type of device. PBS has probably the healthiest programming for your child, and having lived in Alaska (where reception is dodgy) has proven to me that if a person has just one major network channel, that is enough: You can find one or two very satisfying shows each week to concentrate on, and get on with your life doing other things when nothing good is on.

Start group buying and bartering with friends and neighbors. Some friends and I buy and divide up a whole cow or buffalo every few months. As a result, we get the healthiest natural meat for far less than we would pay for the cheapest meat at the supermarket. Other people I know team up to buy local produce from an organic co-op (the weekly basket often contains too much food for a small family, but it could be the right amount if it's split).

Not only is bartering good for establishing community, but is also helpful in localizing your economy, and is great for the environment. Furthermore, bartering is wonderful because you can barter almost anything for anything: Raspberries from your garden for the fresh salmon your neighbor caught, home-made candles for home-made bread... and you can barter services too! Babysitting for window washing, dog walking for car waxing, errand running for tire changes... You may find that tasks that are potentially expensive but too physically draining for you to perform yourself (such as vehicle oil changes) can be performed easily by a neighbor who desperately needs his house cleaned. If you are creative, generous, and honest, you can often find many of your needs met by people in your community of friends and neighbors.

And sometimes there will be that one friend or co-worker who needs or wants nothing in return. Many people in Alaska hunt. Sometimes a friend or friend's husband will hunt a new moose each fall, or would go on a yearly halibut charter, and will get rid of a lot of last year's moose (caribou, salmon, halibut, berries...) because they don't have any room left in their freezer(s). My motto: "I'll take it!" If room in my own the freezer was an issue, I'd find ways to make sure I could take the donation regardless. If it was berries, I'd boil them on the stove, strain them, add lime juice and sugar, and can them in jars in a hot water bath on my stove top. Canning salmon involved more work, time, and a pressure cooker, which might not be your priority to obtain right now, but you get the point. Year-old frozen fish and game meat, unless freezer burned, is still good. Befriend the hunter or the hunter's wife.

Rent out your garage, parking space, or your extra bedroom. If you have a bedroom, garage, or parking space that you don't use, try to get some money for it. Put an ad on Craigslist.org, and screen people well for good credit, etc. Write up a contract, set a firm due date for payment (with a late fee), and always make sure you don't give them the only set of keys to the garage or the only door opener, etc. Renting to the wrong person can make you wish you had never rented—so screen people well to find the right person.

For those of us who have to work:
Some of us will be lucky enough to have the help of friends and relatives during the first few months of our babies' births. However, the reality is that most of us will still have to work in order to meet our needs. Consider these few suggestions in order to possibly free up some of your time.

As you read through suggestions, some may apply to your current reality (working part-time may be feasible for you) and some may not (there's no way you can make a living in your town without working full-time, or you have worked too hard for your specialized education and job to scale back your career involvement). Keep in mind that these are ideas for how you *may* improve your situation and not necessarily recommendations that everyone should explore.

#1: Consider the possibility of finding a part-time that meets your needs. Often times working in a restaurant where you can get great tips can fit the bill. Some jobs consider you a full-time employee and offer company benefits if you work a minimum of 32 hours a week. Sometimes you are in better financial shape working 32 hours a week, as you may still qualify for federal or state medical or child care assistance based on your income, yet you will still be in the workforce—Or you will be paying less for a part-time babysitter than for full-time day care. Always check your county, municipality, or state employment web sites for well-paying part-time jobs. Most people are too caught up in the rat race to even consider a part-time job even if it pays well, but if you have reasonably priced medical care for your baby and your basic needs can be met on a part-time salary, and you are not in a specific evolving career field, there might not be reason to commit forty hours of your time every week.

#2. Consider working at times that your parents or others in your support network can babysit for free or for a reduced amount of pay. For the first few months of my son's life, I temporarily moved in with my parents and found a part-time job that fit their babysitting availability schedule. For me this wasn't a long-term arrangement, but for others it may be.

#3. Strongly consider getting or keeping a job that will allow you to take your baby to work for the first year of his or her life. When my son was an infant, I worked answering phones at a river rafting company where I could set up my son's playpen while I worked, and I can list three companies off the top of my head that have a policy to allow their workers to bring their babies to work with them up to a certain point (usually six months). If you have a long-term relationship with the company you work for, they might be willing to go out on a limb for you during this very vulnerable time, and this can be a tremendous help.

If you have such a situation and still find that your baby greatly reduces your ability to be productive, you may hire a part-time babysitter or child care for one or two days a week—this will help balance your productivity, and the goal is to have both baby and job, not one or the other.

#4. Research low-risk or no-risk work-at-home options. Unless you're already a successful salesperson in such a company, I don't recommend depending entirely on your income from pyramid-marketing type work-at-home opportunities selling cleaning products, makeup, or skin products (and I don't advise venturing into anything that requires more than $100.00 in start-up costs), but there are many work-at-home jobs that provide dependable income. True, there are some scammers out there promising that you can make big money doing practically nothing, which is rarely the case, so keep your antennae up for anything that sounds like a scam, and know that *any* successful work-from-home business is going to require real work.

A more hands-on opportunity: I know a single mom in San Francisco who is the main house cleaner, house-sitter, and dog walker for the people in her apartment building. This has become a great situation because most of her work is conveniently located right in her building, and she rarely has to rush to meet any sort of deadline in order to do a good job and get great referrals. Because she knows that her productivity can depend on the baby, she charges by the job rather than the hour. This creates loyalty from her client/ neighbors.

I also know of a single mom who started a day care business at her home. Only attempt this, however, if you are an extremely patient person with lots of love in her heart for other people's children, childcare experience, and a commitment to do a good job. Also be sure to charge what you're worth. Being in a room with three agitated infants can sometimes make a person go absolutely crazy. Sometimes, however, having a school-aged child or two nearby while you're caring for a baby *can* be a great help. If you take care of infants in your home, make sure you get out with other adults for a couple of hours every weekend.

#5: If you have to work full-time or have an established career occupation and you are attached to staying in your position for whatever reason you have, consider the things you can do to minimize the impact of your separation from your child. Do your best to breastfeed. Co-sleep with your baby whenever possible. Find childcare nearby your office so you can see the baby on your lunch hour (make sure you bring snacks with you and feed yourself during the day—if you don't get enough to eat, your patience will be very thin), or spend a smaller block of time away from the baby. If you have "adult time" at work, it is often easier to commit yourself to your baby when you're not at work.

No matter what you do for a living, save your money diligently during your pregnancy, and take as much maternity leave as you can. As you will see, women deserve to have *paid* maternity leave, so make sure you pay attention to opportunities to speak out, and *always* vote when the political focus is on this very important issue.

◆ ◆ ◆

As I've said before, don't waste a minute of your precious life believing that it's all over. Life changes all the time. If you are ready for (and embrace) these changes, you might find that this nine months of your life was well invested in your happiness and your future, and that your life with your very own child is the best it has ever been. Welcome every day as a new opportunity, and you will be laying the groundwork for a happy, healthy, and fun future for your new little family!

Chapter Eleven

Your Baby Shower

Normally, a book wouldn't go over the details of a baby shower—everyone knows what a baby shower is. But not everyone is depending heavily on getting what they need. Throwing a baby shower is a great way to acquire things that are truly needed, but a bit of planning goes into throwing a successful baby shower. For example, will the shower be thrown at your house or at the home of one of your friends? Would you like to have just one baby shower for all your friends and co-workers, or do you think you should have someone throw you a separate shower at work? Do you want to do all the inviting yourself or have a friend do it? Sometimes there is someone who will volunteer for every necessary task, but sometimes you will have to tie up the loose ends yourself. There are lots of things to consider, so we'll start from the beginning and try to cover all the details.

Finding a host or hostess
Most of the time, an excited friend or family member will volunteer for the task of throwing your baby shower, but if nobody has thought about it, don't be afraid to drop a hint here and there. Sometimes you'll even get a shower for your close personal friends, and a small baby shower at the office as well.

When you finally know who will officially be throwing the shower, let her know who your very best and most dependable friends and family members are so she can delegate a task or two to others within your inner circle. If nobody has offered (which happens sometimes in our busy rat-race culture), throw your own shower.

Finding a site
The best site for having a baby shower is the biggest house you have access to. Still, don't look a gift horse in the mouth if a good friend with a small apartment volunteers to throw you a party. Do ask (without any negative inflection in your voice) how many guests this prospective hostess can handle. If the number seems far lower than you expect, let them know that you wanted to be able to invite X amount of people, but that normally only

60 percent of invited guests show up. See what her reaction is. If her reaction seems negative, tell her you're going to fish around a little more before you'd let her take on such a big responsibility.

Also, many coffee shops and restaurants have "back rooms" or "banquet rooms" that can be rented out for a three-hour party. If space is scarce in your area, maybe this is a way your hostess could make a party work out well.

Establish a time
If you want a traditional three-hour women-only shower, it should probably be held on a weekend afternoon. If instead you want a co-ed shower with beer and silliness, start your shower at five or six and make it a potluck. Always consider the work schedules and other obligations of your prospective guests.

Writing your guest list
Invite everyone you know and everyone you even just kind of know but like. Baby showers rarely get out of control, even if they're very big. Also keep in mind that normally only 25 percent to 60 percent of your invited guests will show, and this will allow you a margin of error. Don't be offended at the people who don't show, just greatly appreciate the ones that do!

Are you one of those women who has lots of male friends? If you are, you might want to make your shower coed. Of course, whether or not to have a coed party depends on you and your group of friends, who is throwing your shower and how traditional they are, etc. Although some single men will pounce on the opportunity to go to a party where their gender is so severely outnumbered, you'll find that most men who would attend such a party are either your friends' husbands, your relatives, and other men who have children and understand what an event it is. Don't expect a large number of men you invite to attend—just be thankful and appreciative if they do, and make sure there's enough activity to keep them from getting bored.

Invitations
It is very important that you get your invitations out *early*. You should allow for at least three weeks so that your friends can clear their schedules. These days, it is far cheaper to send invitations electronically, and probably most efficient and cheapest to set up the party on Facebook or some other social media site so people can get reminders and see the event updates in their news feed. Remember there are also people you will want to invite who are not your Facebook friends, or people who just aren't into social media, so make sure you get a few traditional paper invitations as well. It is wise to include a

stamped envelope addressed to the hostess or an email address for the hostess so that your friends can RSVP (or so that they can send a gift if they cannot attend). This way your hostess can prepare for the amount of guests, although sometimes people show up who have not responded.

Your invitations should always include the name and address of your hostess or host site (both physical address and directions or a clear map), the phone number of the hostess, and the gender of the baby (if known), or a request for unisex clothing, etc., if you plan to keep the gender a surprise.

There is some argument as to whether or not it is proper to include where the baby's mother is registered for gifts. Although the "old school" method is to leave this information out with the assumption that the guests will call the hostess and ask, we can't always depend on our guests knowing the system. I chose to include this information on my invitations. A friend of mine did not, and was inundated with things she couldn't use and couldn't return. The choice is yours.

Registering for your baby shower

Most department stores with a baby department will have a baby shower registry. Registering for your baby shower is a great way of familiarizing yourself with some things you never knew existed and assuring that your guests will know which brands you prefer and will be most likely to use. Sometimes the breadth of items available will be overwhelming—not everything that is listed on shower registries is something that is necessary, so make sure you get your priorities straight. Also, when registering, keep in mind the incomes of your invited guests. Make sure you register for the little things you want as well as the big things so that your friends can feel good about what they bought you even if they don't have much money. Sometimes people surprise you by teaming up to buy you something really grand, so don't neglect to register for *some* of the high-ticket items even if you don't have wealthy guests.

Also remember that women like to buy clothes! You may end up with surprisingly little in the area of necessities and a substantial enough wardrobe to have the best-dressed baby in town. Whether you plan to return the clothes and use the cash for something necessary or plan to take the less frequently used items to a consignment or a buy-sell-trade store when the baby outgrows them is your business, but always show appreciation for what you get whether you like or need it or don't.

Hand-outs, games and activities, and door prizes

Always give back to the people who are giving to you. Here are some ideas to help show your guests that they are appreciated and cherished for being your guests.

Hand-Outs

Every good shower has something special for the guests, but most baby shower party favors are useless things like rattles and tiny over-priced plastic dolls. I would personally recommend something more adult-oriented. After all, *you're* the one having the baby, not them. What do *they* need with a little rattle? Instead, reward your steadfast friends with inexpensive hand-outs like packs of incense, lip balms, bubble-gum cigars that say "It's a boy" or "It's a girl," candles, perfume or makeup samples (easy to obtain if you or the hostess works in a department store), and so on.

Making it Memorable

Activities are also a very important part of making a memorable baby shower. I was recently at a co-ed shower during which guests were asked to dress up as (and act like) the mother and father of the baby being born, were awarded for the most accurate portrayal, and the whole event was captured on video. In addition, the hostess and her friends got together and made a comedy film about giving birth and showed it at the shower. That has been the most unforgettable baby shower I have attended to date.

Another great idea is to have guests bring home-made frozen meals for the mother-to-be in addition to baby shower gifts. This gives your friends and family the opportunity to show off their favorite recipes and takes the strain off the mother-to-be to go out and buy food if she's up and hungry in the middle of the night (which she will be). Guests can assemble their recipes in the disposable aluminum bread pans that can be acquired cheaply at the supermarket (one on the bottom and one on the top to cover it, secured with a rubber band), ingredients can be listed on the aluminum container with a sharpie pen (be sure to include the date the meal was prepared). The meal can be frozen in the bread pans and brought to the shower. The mother-to-be (that's *you*) can thaw it, heat it up, and eat it within a few weeks.

Your hostess may have her own ideas about what games she wants to play at your baby shower, but following are three examples of simple traditional games to assure that you and your guests are entertained.

1: The M&M in the diaper game
   Fold tissues into diaper shapes and squirt a small dab of yellow mustard in one of the diapers and put an M&M in one. Have the guests pick the diapers from a bowl. The guest who gets the M&M diaper wins a door prize.
2: Baby Shower Bingo
   This game works best if you have lots of people attending your shower: Make bingo cards (all of them different) with the names of the most common items that you included on your registry in each space. Have your guests fill out their bingo

cards while you unwrap your presents. Whoever gets to bingo first acquires a prize. You can make this a continuing game if you like, but if you do, make sure the door prizes are simple and inexpensive.

3: How Big is Mama?

Have everybody take a piece of yarn that they think represents the biggest part of your belly. After everyone has guessed, you take a piece of string and measure yourself. He or she who comes closest to your measurements wins a prize.

Door Prizes

Again, it is important that you don't go broke acquiring door prizes for your guests. If your shower is coed, make sure that the prizes are things that will be useful to the men as well as the women, and if children are invited, remember that (for some reason) kids seem to do very well with contests and games. For this reason, gift cards are highly recommended.

Refreshments

Always make sure that refreshments are provided at your baby shower. A good variety of snacks would include cake, punch, finger foods, veggie sticks and dip, and depending on your guests and the time of day of the shower, maybe wine or champagne for those who are not pregnant.

A good way to take pressure off the hostess is to have the party be a potluck. Everyone gets to bring something they know how to make and are proud of. Let your hostess know which of your friends seems to have the most enthusiasm, and let them know which appetizers which friends have brought to parties in case a little "Mari says your broccoli salad is to die for" schmooze is in order. However, be careful of overkill (or over-ask). Don't have a potluck *and* implement the frozen food idea. Many people may lose the spirit of having fun helping you if they feel overworked. Design your shower to provide a balance for your guests. You want them to have fun.

Thank You Cards

Designate a friend to write down what you received and from whom while you are opening your gifts. Make sure you thank everyone for their contributions to your baby's welfare. If you're soon to deliver your baby, everyone will understand if they don't get their cards right away, but make certain that you don't forget completely, as some people are very offended by this.

With all these factors considered, your shower is sure to be a success. It is natural to be a bit frazzled and wonder if everyone is having a good time, but don't let yourself get worn out or distracted. Remember that you and your little baby are the guests of honor, and that it is your guests' duty to come up and acknowledge you, not vice versa. Try to spend some quality time with each of the guests you haven't seen in a while, but keep in mind that everyone will understand that you are trying your best to be a good guest of honor.

Chapter Twelve

Birthing Your Way

You may have noticed that I, as an author, have focused on the sociology of being single, pregnant, and happy rather than the mechanics of pregnancy and childbirth. There are several reasons for this: First of all, I am not a childbirth educator or childbirth professional—I I am merely a single mother who went through something similar to what you are going through, I am always glad I followed through with my decision, and I became an advocate for people like myself. I feel that the job of educating you on the mechanics of childbirth belongs with those professionals who have dedicated years of their lives to the study and practice of childbirth.

Secondly, I feel that it is my primary responsibility to honor your free will regarding the decisions that can impact you for the rest of your life. I realize that just because something has worked for me does not necessarily mean that it will work for you. As you can probably tell, I'm a pretty strong supporter of doing things the "natural" way, and my history as a food safety and security activist (as well as my years of parenting an allergic child) has helped me to develop some strong opinions about those government bodies that regulate healthcare, food safety, and social services. But who am I, and who is anyone else to tell you what is truly best for you when we haven't walked in your shoes?

Some people cringe at the idea of having a home birth, and some people cringe at the idea of a scheduled C-Section. I do have to admit that my prenatal care and my son's hospital birth left a *lot* to be desired (my intended natural birth ended up including forceps), but I've been assured by some women who birthed at home or in birthing centers that they too were not provided with the personalized and caring support that they expected from their midwives.

On the other hand, I have known people who have had completely positive experiences with whichever option ultimately resulted in a healthy baby.

Whether you have a positive or negative birth experience will depend on so many factors that it is impossible to say that there is a "right" way or a "wrong" way to give birth, as right and wrong are all relative to she who is going through the experience, and are of course strongly related to whether or not the baby comes through it all right.

What is most important to me is that you are happy, healthy, emotionally stable, and provide the best life for your child that you can. I must admit that my motives are extremely selfish: It might be *your* son who ends up being the manager at the senior housing facility that I live in when I'm eighty. Do I want to be cared for by a person who is happy, healthy, secure, and loves his mother? Or do I want to be cared for by someone with major issues and resentments? I have no way of proving this to myself or anyone else, but I feel that happiness, fulfillment, and emotional stability can be achieved regardless of whatever trauma a person experiences in birth, although it is known that some mothers and babies have needed healing for extremely traumatic experiences.

That said, I am going to stick to facts rather than opinions. Keep in mind that there may be some truths that I fail to discuss, but I am going to leave those truths in the hands of whichever childbirth educator you decide to put your faith in.

My adherence to the principal of honoring your free will is the result of having been judged, having witnessed judgment, having seen the negative impacts of judgment, and even having done some unfair judging myself. I have known some women who adhered to the highest natural parenting standards who were belittled and ridiculed by their peers because their intended natural births ultimately resulted in C-sections. ("You didn't try hard enough. Your decision was selfish. You have ultimately failed your child.") I have known some women whose neighbors, friends and even their mothers disowned them because they disagreed with these women's choices to give birth in their homes ("How irresponsible of you! That's a horrible, selfish, and dangerous decision. I totally disagree with what you are doing."). A relative of mine chose to have a scheduled C-section because of a serious heart condition that was diagnosed in her youth. She could hardly get the word "scheduled" out of her mouth without sending people stomping off in disapprobation. Another friend opted for a C-section, *upon the advice of her midwife*, because her baby was both breach and her umbilical cord was wrapped twice around her neck. She too was used as a negative example while attending a postnatal yoga class. Back in the late sixties, my mother endured harsh judgment from her friends, neighbors, and even her doctors, for exercising when she was pregnant, opting for natural childbirth, and breastfeeding. It seems like no matter what you do, *someone* will be determined to have a problem with it!

But that's their problem, not yours. And I find it so odd that all these people claim to have such compassion for the babies, but seemingly no compassion at all for the babies' mothers, and no understanding for the diversity and potential complexity in their individual situations.

At one point I was approached by a well-known author and childbirth educator who wished to add birthing information to my book. I thought that would be a great idea, as my knowledge only went as far as my personal experience—which was one of impersonal bad service, medical drama, and subsequent financial ruin—I was in no way an authority on how to have a good birth experience, so I thought I'd let her help. After investing some time on the re-write, I grew tired of her assertion that mothers who did not strictly adhere to her ideas of what is a healthy birth experience will produce babies who will be, in her own words, "fucked up." In her opinion, the fact that my own son is an honor student, a great athlete, and loves his mother with all his heart will all be canceled out one day when he is barraged with a storm of bitterness and anger because I hadn't "pushed hard enough." She felt that I needed to embrace and fully feel the "guilt" of having failed myself and my child, and she felt that embracing this guilt was something that should be encouraged for my audience, which completely goes against everything I stand for.

It should be noted that, for the most part, childbirth educators are extremely loving, helpful, and compassionate people. When all was said and done, it was easy to see that this particular woman's life and choices provided no example to follow, as she was of the school of thought that the number one priority of a single mother should be to become un-single as soon as possible, and that my "failure" to find the appropriate partner over the last few years was not a result of high standards and holding out for the right chemistry, but was instead a result of some deep wound that kept me angry at men. Of course I had no defense—I don't carry pictures of all the men in my life in my wallet. I don't move through every moment of every day feeling inadequate because I haven't encountered my one and only. She has her own truth, and I'll let her keep it.

But just like she has her truth and I have mine, you have yours. In order to make sure that your truth is yours and yours alone, listen to *yourself*. Follow your own heart and your own instincts. Do your own research on birthing and parenting options. Don't let anybody else's fears or issues dictate what it is you need to do. Exercise your own values, refrain from judging anyone else for their choices, and refrain from judging yourself in the event that your change your mind or fail to follow through with what you had originally planned. The "should," "can," and "will" of your situation are all up to you, and you deserve the privilege of making your own decisions.

Birthing Options
You have lots of options for how you want to give birth, but whether a birthing option holds appeal will depend entirely on your personal life experience and individual priorities. Birthing options range from Scheduled C-Sections to Emergency C-Sections, to induced labor to births with Epidurals, births with forceps and suction devices, to births with local anesthetic, to natural childbirth in hospitals to natural childbirth in birthing centers and homes, unassisted births, water births, hypno-births, silent births, and if you have a high budget and the right connections, you can even give birth in a dolphin tank! Did I miss anything? I'm sure I did. Unless you constantly have your finger on the pulse

of birthing, it's impossible to know all of the available options. Talk to your midwife or doctor about what is available to you for your budget.

Doctor or Midwife?
Again, whether to opt for a midwife or a doctor is a matter of personal preference. Women who are committed to following through with natural childbirth and would like personalized service can often find the service they want in a midwife. Midwives are often far less expensive than doctors, they often require far fewer check-ups if things seem to going smoothly, and despite what you may have been told, some midwives can be reimbursed through Medicaid. Others are licensed and certified to give birth in hospitals, or to remain at your side in the event that unforeseen complications arise that require medical care. Some first-time moms like the option of giving birth at a birth center nearby the hospital in case such complications arise.

Doctors often provide less personalized care, and required prenatal visits are often costly. Sometimes a "patient" visits the Ob-GYN office several times before she even meets her doctor, and often times, their babies are not even delivered by their doctor, but are instead delivered by another doctor in the doctor's group. This can be a big deal to some people. However, depending on your medical history (especially in the event that you are taking certain medications, etc.) and your level of apprehension about giving birth, this may be the option you feel is best for you.

Regardless of whether you ultimately choose a doctor or a midwife, the care provider you choose should be someone who listens to you, answers your questions, respects your priorities, and cares about your situation. If at any point you are dissatisfied with the care you are receiving, don't be afraid to *fire them* and move on.

When I was pregnant, I was treated as though I was the biggest hypochondriac in the world. Throughout my own pregnancy, I only had one complication: I had an extremely painful condition which I have since learned was interstitial cystitis, but at the time I was treated as though I had a bladder infection, urinary tract infection, or a kidney infection. According to my doctor, we needed to find out "what kind" of infection I had. At first she opted to put me on antibiotics. If that didn't work within a week, there was another option that could be exercised, but we had to try the antibiotics first.

While in the extremely painful throes of this infection during that week of failed diagnosis, I was called in for jury duty. I explained to the woman who was working with jury selection that I couldn't perform due to having to go to the bathroom frequently because I was pregnant and had an infection. She said that I needed to supply a written statement from my doctor that I had this urinary infection.

Within the three days that I attempted to contact my doctor, none of my calls were returned. In order to speak to my doctor, I had to schedule an appointment (which I needed to do anyway, as the antibiotics were clearly not providing me with any relief). When I finally got a chance to see my doctor, she told me she would rather not excuse me from jury duty because pregnancy wasn't in and of itself reason enough to get out of my responsibility, even though I was in pain from my infection. Thankfully, despite her refusal to write a letter for me, I instead submitted a copy of my bill to the court, which sufficed as proof of my discomfort. On the day of my son's birth (which was, by the way, his due date) my doctor was not available to deliver my son, but I didn't mind. I preferred the doctor who delivered my son, even though I'd never even met him.

Although some might feel that my experience lends itself to selecting a midwife instead of an Ob-GYN, midwives also need to be thoroughly screened for professionalism. A friend of mine said that it was "like pulling teeth" to get her midwife to return her calls (even though she'd had some potentially dangerous bleeding spells), and honor her appointments (she missed several of them). The only requests that this friend made were to 1) have access to a birthing tub, and 2) to be given birthing classes in her home, as she lived in a rural setting and didn't want to drive far in order to learn how to give birth. The birthing classes were never performed, and the birthing tub was in the possession of a different midwife when my friend needed it.

On the day that my friend gave birth, this midwife treated her as though she didn't know what she was talking about when she called to announce that she was in labor, and arrived several hours after the baby had been successfully delivered by the friend's husband and an apprentice who was not yet legal to catch the baby. However, this friend was extremely happy with her birth experience, as she felt that the universe had empowered her to give birth practically unassisted. I, on the other hand, was angry to hear that my friend didn't even know what it meant when the apprentice told her to "push." It was her *husband* (the son of a retired midwife) who had cleared up this understanding by telling her to "push as though you're having a bowel movement." This misunderstanding wouldn't have happened if she had been given the birthing classes she had requested.

But just as you can receive substandard service, there are lots of winners out there too. In my opinion, whether your caregiver will or will not make you happy will depend largely on the service you are given. Following are a few questions to ask your caregiver that will help you to nail down the right one.

If you prefer to give birth with the assistance of a Midwife
Some women are determined to give birth without any medical intervention whatsoever, and some women like knowing that the option of medical intervention is available if it's needed. Ask your midwife about her philosophy and make sure her philosophy matches yours.

If you prefer the prenatal care of a midwife but want the reassurance of medical intervention if necessary (or desired, depending on your philosophy), ask your midwife whether she's licensed and willing to remain with you in the event that medical intervention is chosen.

Look carefully at your contract, and discuss it with your midwife. Some midwives who work tandem with doctors might request full payment for her services even if she doesn't deliver (or receive) your baby. This might be fine with you if she remains with you throughout your labor, but you might honestly not have enough money to pay for a midwife and a doctor if you're "handed off" to an Ob-Gyn. Talk about this with your midwife.

One of the great things about midwives (and Doulas, which are professional birthing assistants) is that they often provide a multitude of services along with their practice: massage therapy and other types of body work and energy work, childbirth education, post-natal lactation consulting, etc. See what kind of extra services are offered in your midwife's standard contract.

Most of all, make sure you like her. Make sure she respects your decisions, and don't be frightened or let yourself be pressured into taking any path that does not completely resonate with you. Midwives are individuals, and you can certainly find one who understands your needs and desires, whatever they may be.

If you prefer to give birth with the assistance of an Ob-Gyn
Make sure your doctor seems to be on *your* side and respects your priorities. If, for example, you are leaning towards doing things as naturally as possible, do not let your doctor "talk (you) out of" doing what your heart is telling you to do. If they speak about risks and complications associated with taking a certain path, make sure they are specific and tell you what those risks are.

Make sure your doctor is available to you. If you have questions, either your doctor or someone in her office should have the time and energy to give you an answer that satisfies you. If not, there is no harm in finding another, no matter how far along you are in your pregnancy. Don't be a pain in the ass, and be patient, but don't take any crap from anyone.

No matter which you choose
I have met pushy midwives and pushy doctors. Of course, I have also met doctors and midwives who are very understanding and want to make sure that your birth experience is everything that you want it to be, and will be honest with you about the benefits and drawbacks of any particular choice. In my opinion, a good caregiver is one that is not polarized. He or she realizes that every situation is a combination of circumstances, and that there is no one-size-fits-all solution.

Remember that for some people, birth is a business: The more services they sell you, the more money they can make. Our society really did us a disservice when they touted medicine and law as the big "money making" professions. What did we get? Corrupt doctors, and corrupt lawyers. But always remember that *you* are the boss. You are the one paying for their service—it is their job to give you what you ask for, not insist that you do things their way. Sometimes, believe it or not, if you educate yourself well, you might know more about a particular topic than your caregiver!

Take for example my son's pediatrician: He was a good man who had been practicing for decades, and had applauded me for choosing not to circumcise my son—in his own words, to leave my son intact was more "natural." However, he had recommended an infant formula that I later found to contain genetically engineered ingredients and growth hormones. He had been recommending this formula to all his patients for years. When I told him that the formula he had been recommending contained GMOs, he asked, "What's a GMO?"

Remember that a caregiver has a job and you have yours. Doctors are good for doing things you can't do: administering drugs, performing surgery, and diagnosing certain conditions. Same goes for midwives—you can't really give yourself a massage, your probably don't have everything you need to make a belly cast, and are not aware of all the ways you can maximize the safety and enjoyment of your birth experience. That is their service to you. Make sure they fulfill it and don't overstep into your personal decisions.

The Big Day
When it comes to getting ready for the big day, there's really not much to it—and if you tackle all those little tasks ahead of time, the day itself can be appreciated more fully if you know what to expect from the hospital or birth center, and you know what you need to do for yourself. Here are some suggestions to help assure the ease of those logistical matters in your big event.

1. It is imperative that you have arrangements for transportation to the hospital or birth center. If you don't have solid arrangements or if your transportation falls through, call a taxi or an ambulance if you need one!
2. Don't forget to commission a friend or relative with a flexible schedule to take you home after the birth of your baby or to bring you your car.
3. Make a list of those people who want to be notified when you are going into labor, and a separate list of those who want to be notified when the baby is born, and put it in your birthing suitcase or smartphone (if you are birthing away from home).

4. If you have your own car, make sure you properly install your baby's car seat well ahead of time—not only is it the law, but it is very necessary, even if you don't get caught without one.
5. If you have pets, plants, other children, or other household obligations, arrange for their care ahead of time, and make sure your sitters can honor your request at a moment's notice and can assist on an open-ended schedule in case you have complications that keep you or your baby in the hospital or birth center for longer than you had planned.

Aside from that, the only thing you will need to prepare is your suitcase, which should be packed far ahead of time for obvious reasons.

Packing Your Suitcase

You may be surprised at what you will or won't need while you are in the birth center or hospital. You might want to wear your own nightgown while you are in labor, but despite the potentially unflattering style, it's best to use the gown provided if you give birth in the hospital—after all, labor can be a real mess! The only major drawback to the hospital's gown is that it will have opening flaps for your breasts, which are unnecessary while you are in labor (but will come in handy shortly thereafter), and you may want to assign a girlfriend to "modesty check" if you have male friends in the room while you are in early labor, as these flaps have a tendency to "flap" open.

Throughout your pregnancy, you will read many lists of what you will need in the birth center, but a person's true needs will vary widely from one individual to the next. Following is a list of what I found necessary while I was in labor and in the hospital thereafter. Please note that while many of these things are likely on your smartphone, there may still be a reader or two who doesn't have one for financial reasons or lifestyle choices, or readers who don't realize their phones have these capabilities because they've never used them).

> Phone/Smartphone
> Robe
> Slippers
> Lip Balm
> Makeup
> Lotion
> Skin care products
> Scented oil or natural perfume (after the big event you will feel as if you smell like a farm animal)

Hair Brush
Camera (if you don't have a smartphone)
Hairstyling necessities
Two or more nightgowns or nursing gowns (that you are not afraid of receiving guests and being photographed in
Two or more bras or nursing bras if you plan to breast feed (a cup size larger than before)
Nursing breast pads if you plan to breast feed
List of people to notify
Toothbrush & Paste
Going Home Outfit (second trimester size)
Going Home Outfit and Blanket for Baby
Car Seat for Baby
Watch (if you don't have a smartphone)
Contact lens case and glasses
Calendar or appointment book (if you don't have a smartphone)
Book or magazine
Folder to store scraps, first photo, paperwork, footprints, etc.

If you have a birthing coach, she or he may want to bring certain things along as well not only for her (or his) own comfort for what may be a long haul, but to help the time pass for you as well.

As for necessary items to help you, these may or may not include:

iPod or Mp3 player with your favorite music
Watch with second hand
Massage oil and items for back massage
Fan
Camera
Extra Pillows
Board games or playing cards

Although it seems as though many people put a lot of time and energy into preparing for childbirth, the truth is that it's going to take its course no matter how well or how badly you have prepared for it. If you find yourself in a situation in which you must rush to the birth center or hospital without your go-bag, try not to worry too much, as these places will roughly meet your basic needs. It is still best to be prepared, as the prices of personal items in the hospital is normally very high and the selection disappointing, but if all else fails, you can always ask a friend to run home and get your bag (people like to have an important role), or commission (beg) a staff member to run to the gift store and get what you need.

That said, starting a month before your due date, as yourself weekly: Am I ready? Where's my bag? Is the kitchen stocked? Have I done everything that needs to be done? Are you sure? Okay then, away you go. You'll have the time of your life!

Battle Scars and Bragging Rights
It is only natural for us to feel fear when we are stepping into the unknown, but the fact remains that your birth experience will likely be remembered as a positive experience.

My personal experience started when my water broke. I was watching *Mary Poppins*, and I got the feeling of a rubber band being snapped in my stomach with a weird "thunk" noise. Within a few seconds, I knew what had happened: My water broke. As I was getting ready for the ride to the hospital, Igor, my parents' boxer, came into my room and saw the water leaking out of me and onto the floor. His eyes bugged out as if to say, "You're going to get in *big* trouble for peeing on the floor!"

I didn't even realize I was having contractions when I arrived at the hospital. The first contractions merely felt like mild menstrual cramps (keep in mind that everybody's experience is different). I only realized that they were indeed contractions when the nurses hooked me up to monitors and were surprised that I didn't feel much of anything. My mother's birth experiences had been, in her words, practically painless (and I don't disbelieve her, as this is indeed the claim that many women make), and I wondered if I would be afforded the same luck. But no, that didn't last.

When I walked from the triage room to the delivery room, that's when it happened. The feeling was still a lot like menstrual cramps, except it was a thousand (Million? Billion?) times stronger. I had the overwhelming urge to squat and deposit all of that fiery pain into the ground below me. I forgot all about my own head and feet, and just became one big, painful yawning belly-mass. It was intense.

Painful as it was, I just managed from minute to minute until it was all over. I didn't do anything I was "supposed" to do. I didn't breathe right, I didn't look at my birth in the mirror to keep me calm and focused, I didn't *care* if I remained calm and focused, and I didn't do anything the doctor and nurses asked me to do—it took eight people to hold me down. I just wanted to get up and *run for my life*! Of course, I couldn't run anywhere to get away from it all, but try telling that to someone who is in so much pain that they can't even think. I screamed like a torture victim, I talked back to the nurses, I rebelled, I peed the bed… oh well. In came the doctor, out came the forceps, and then I knew this was not going to be a typical birth experience. I sat up three times asking the doctor different questions to try and stall him. I didn't want those forceps, but my desire to get it over with ultimately eclipsed my fear of pain. I finally accepted what was to happen and just cooperated with the doctor. A minute of forceps, and my son was out.

After my son was born, I apologized to the doctor and nurses for my behavior. They just shrugged. "No big deal," they said. "We've seen it all."

I guess my point is, no matter what you do or don't do right, the baby is going to come out one way or another! Some people will go round and round about the "right way" to do things. Some people have asserted that a "traumatic" birth such as mine requires healing. But the truth for me is that I wouldn't have had it any other way: It was a big release, and after all I'd been through, there was a lot of screaming that just needed to come out of me. The process in itself was healing enough. If I give birth again, it will be different, but I don't resent that day. My beautiful boy came out that day! How could anything I underwent be not perfect? If I have another child, the experience will be much more calm, but I won't say that such an experience is "better" than what I went through with my son. To me, it seems fitting that our amazing life together would begin with a primal scream.

Hours later, I found myself bragging to all my friends about how it took three people to hold each leg down and how I screamed perpetually for five minutes and my mother wondered if I had been possessed by a spirit. All the pain and fear was gone, and I had a great story to tell!

So no matter what does or does not happen in your own birth experience, it'll be like your own very personal carnival ride that you'll never forget, filled with excitement and heroism. You've already proven to yourself and your loved ones that you are a strong, independent woman. The event of your child's birth will prove it to the world!

Secrets of Navigating a Hospital Birth

If you do opt to give birth in a hospital, here are a few tidbits you may or may not have known about your hospital stay, facts that may make your stay easier or less expensive than if you hadn't known them.

Medical professionals often recommend that you stay in the hospital for three days. Why do they do that? Who knows? Women who give birth at home don't stay at the hospital for three days. If money is an issue, you have a healthy baby, and have support at home, I say go home right after you've had a nice, long nap.

For some strange reason, it costs a *lot* more to take the pain medications the nurse gives you than it does to have your doctor write you out a prescription and have a friend retrieve them from the pharmacy. If you have no one at your disposal, have a nice and agreeable nurse run and pick up the scrip for you. If nobody is willing to help you, cry if you have to. Make a nuisance of yourself. Do what you must. Just don't pay seventy dollars for three doses of medication when a whole bottle costs you ten.

You will be charged for every sanitary pad, ointment, diaper, baby wipe, nasal aspirator, and ice pack in your room, and you'll be surprised to find how much they charge for such things: a box of sanitary pads at the hospital will set you back about forty bucks! If you get a chance to haggle your bill, be sure to point these things out. Normally these bills just go to insurance companies, and they have the money to pay this, but *you* are not an insurance company! Don't wait for anyone to notice this. Be polite, but speak up!

Whether you ultimately pay for these things or not, these charges will appear on your bill even if you don't take the stuff, as they're supposed to be thrown out for sanitary reasons if you don't, so take everything that isn't nailed down, even if you don't think you'll need it.

You will encounter both good and bad nurses while in the hospital. Nursing is a very labor-intensive job, and burnout is rather common. If you feel that you are not receiving the care you expect, you may request a different nurse, but don't be *too* demanding or you may be ignored when you need help.

Although you've often heard it said that nothing can compete with the feeling a woman gets when she first holds her baby in her arms, if you don't feel bonded with your baby right away, there is nothing wrong with you. Many women admit that they didn't "know" their child right away, and didn't feel bonded until the child's personality emerged at two or three months of age. It is more likely that you'll feel an immediate bond with your child if you come from a large family with lots of babies or if you've always yearned for a child of your own, but if you find yourself surprised at the separation you feel from your newborn, try to think of him as a doll who needs constant and gentle care until something happens that shows you that he is a very special little human that you've created with comparatively little help from anyone else.

Although situations vary from woman to woman, I didn't feel bonded with my son for about eleven weeks. I did love him, and I was very protective of this strange little creature I had made, but the true connection didn't happen until he started interacting with me. If you feel alienated from your baby, be patient, and give yourself a break. In time you'll know him and understand his role in your life.

Don't feel guilty if you have to leave your baby in the nursery for a few hours so that you can rest. Sleep will be in short supply for a stretch of time, so take advantage of the opportunity to sleep deeply.

One nurse had implied that I was shirking my responsibilities when I hadn't seen my son since his birth, five hours earlier. It was ten in the morning, and I had stayed up all night. As you can imagine, it was weeks before I got caught up on the sleep I missed from that very evening. I wish she hadn't successfully pressured me into cutting my sleep short, because it's so hard to be happy and excited when you're exhausted. As I've said before, you've got to be your own best friend.

Lactation consultants can be a big help if you are breastfeeding, and they can also be a big pain in the ass regardless of whether or not you're breastfeeding. If you need their help, let them in and let them help you. If you don't need their help, don't hesitate to tell them to go away.

♦ ♦ ♦

I hope these suggestions will help save you time, money, and stress before, after, and during on the date of your new arrival and the few days following.

If you opt for a hospital birth, Do your best to keep your head on straight from the moment you arrive at the hospital, and you will have a better chance of knowing where your money will go and what's going on with you and your baby.

If you opt for a birth in a birthing center, in your home, or any other site, make sure you have a midwife and /or support staff that you are completely comfortable with and have faith in.

I wish you the best of luck, with knowledge that it will all work out great!

Chapter Thirteen

Into Your Near Future as a Single Mom

Once your newborn is home, you may be overwhelmed with the amount of work and responsibility that comes along with having your baby. True, it is a lot of work, but anything is manageable if you have the right attitude. The first rule of new single motherhood is this: *Make life easy on yourself.* Following are a few tips on how this can be done.

Help yourself to a few weeks of leave from your job.
If maternity leave is paid, great! If not, take it anyway. If your job has more than 50 employees in your area, they must allow you up to 12 week unpaid maternity leave through FMLA. Some states have supplemented these regulations with additional benefits. As you will see, you will need this time to adjust to your new life and to take care of both of you. You can use this time to research child care options, apply for Day Care Assistance, and show off your baby to everyone who hasn't seen him yet. Furthermore your body will take a couple weeks to shrink back down to a stable size, and you may want to pack up the baby and introduce him to the mall to get some clothes that you can wear in the slim-down transition.

Get yourself organized ahead of time.
Before the baby is born, stock up on everything you are certain you will need, including non-perishable food items, diapers, baby wipes, laundry soap, etc. It will not be easy to jet out at a moment's notice and get what you need during those first weeks, so stock up as though you're waiting for Armageddon. If you or a friend has a membership at Costco or Sam's Club, now is the time to plan a visit to the price club.

Try to get someone to help you for the first two weeks or more.
If you have a friend or relative who will help you, consider yourself lucky. It is highly recommended to have a friend, relative, or a revolving combination of both stay with you for

the first six weeks (or longer) of your baby's life. Depending on your life circumstances, you might want to temporarily (or semi-permanently) move in with your parents. When my son was born, I moved in with my parents and rented out a condo I owned so I wouldn't have to worry about paying rent or having a place to go to when I felt it was time to have my independent life back.

If you don't have such options, you might want to hire a temporary nanny (with newborn experience) to either watch the baby while you tend to your errands or to help with housework. Depending on your area, you may have access to social programs that will send a helper to your home, or that will provide emergency child care for women who are about to pull their hair out.

Catholic Social Services in your area may be able to refer you to such programs. Research whether there is such a program in your area—if there is, take advantage of it, and don't feel bad about doing what you have to do to stay sane. Use the time to catch up on sleep, clean your house, or even dress up and go out with friends. Use it to do whatever you can't do with the baby along for the ride, whatever you think is going to make your job as a working single mother easier, and don't feel guilty about it. Even mothers with husbands and nannies feel like they're going crazy sometimes, so you should not feel the least bit ashamed for giving yourself a break. Yes, there are people who abuse such programs, go on benders, drop their kids off every week, and obviously have the wrong priorities—but don't let that stop you from doing what needs to be done. Remember that there are times that it is also in your child's best interests that you take a break, so it's for the baby too.

Don't be afraid to let a healthy baby cry for short periods of time.
Although nobody wants to let a baby cry, and every attempt should be made to find out why a baby is crying and to comfort him, there are times in a single mother's life when it's necessary to let a baby cry for a short amount of time. When you get up in the morning, after the baby is fed and changed, if any task is too difficult to complete with the baby in a sling, put the baby down long enough to wash your own face, brush your teeth, dress, and eat. Allow yourself two or three ten-minute breaks a day to get yourself squared away. This will help you to be more ready when you are able to give the baby attention, and then you'll be better able either to rest or get the lower-priority tasks taken care of when the baby is sleeping.

And as I've said before and will say again, a baby monitor is absolutely necessary. If you need to step out into the sunshine and breathe, and the only way to do so is to go out three security exits, you must do what you must do in order to remain sane. Be sure to attach all your necessary house keys to the baby monitor, and don't rely on it for any longer than five minutes (it's not a babysitter).

Give Yourself Time to (ahem) "Normalize"

Yes, you may be extremely discomfited by the changes in your body after you've had a baby. You will still look pregnant for up to a few weeks after you've had the baby, and some might even assume that you are *still* pregnant, not realizing that the baby in your stroller is the one you pushed out three weeks ago. Don't be offended—some people just don't know.

Another story that may be of interest: I had been told that it would take six weeks for certain parts of my anatomy (okay, I'm talking about my vagina) to shrink back down to a normal size after giving birth. At my six-week checkup, when the doctor put the speculum in my vagina and scraped my cervix, I couldn't feel a thing—everything down there was loose and numb. "What a dirty trick," I thought to myself, "for them to tell us that we wouldn't be stretched out for the rest of our lives." I likened it to when the doctor gives you a shot and tells you it's not going to hurt: just another medical lie. At that moment I said to myself, "well, *that*'s ruined, so I guess I've got to accept myself for what I am *now* and move on." Once while the two of us were complaining about how our bodies had changed, a friend of mine who is an avid jogger volunteered that she had peed in her pants every time she'd gone jogging since her daughter was born.

It just so happens that my "nether regions" did indeed make a complete recovery (as did those of my jogger friend), but it took far longer than six weeks. Everybody's time frame is different, so don't get discouraged, frightened, or depressed if your body hasn't recovered within the "normal" time frame.

The Myth of Postnatal Glamour

Despite the fact that the whole world seems obsessed with new motherhood, the fact is it is not exactly a bed of roses for most of us—after all, sleep deprivation, a sparseness of opportunity to concentrate on anything, and the scarcity of time to improve your appearance or clean your house is about enough to drive anyone freaky. I remember admiring all the beautiful clothes and toys people had bought me for my son and thinking, "no matter how it looks when it stands alone, it still looks like crap when it smells like spit-up and is wadded up in a huge pile on the floor." I out-and-out resented our culture's attachment to pastel colors for babies because they show stains so much worse than bright or dark colors.

Yes, the "glamour" of new motherhood is another factor that proves most people are living in unreality, and the idea that your little angel baby is going to fill your heart with joy every moment of every day is another whopper of a lie we're told, which may in turn make us feel "wrong" or "bad" in the event that we don't immediately feel this strong loving bond with our babies. If you struggle with moments of "this isn't at all what I thought it would be," that's okay. We are all human, and are better able to take care of others if we ourselves are taken care of first.

My Difficult Baby

Before my son was born, my mother had said, "There's no feeling that can compete with the first moment your child looks into your eyes with such love…" She'd also said, "If a baby is crying, it's because his needs are not being met. You and your sister were the best babies. You never cried."

Well, when MY son first looked into my eyes, his expression was more like, "Ew, what's *that*?" As a matter of fact, my son didn't smile at me or look at me with any expression other than a sneer for about the first three months of his life. His every waking moment was spent either screaming or crying. If I ever tried to snuggle up with him, he'd scream and pull my hair. I swore the kid hated me! It wasn't until he was about six months old that he seemed to like me (although *he* seems to "remember" loving me always, so it's important not to assume anyone else's feelings. When I joke about his apparent dislike of me and preference for his grandma during that time, he insists that I was mistaken). Throughout those first six months of caring for my "not-so-sweet" baby, I was certain I had given birth to his father's child and not my own, and I suspected that he was going to be a troubled child and we would always have a strained relationship. Sadly, the observations of friends, strangers, and caregivers seemed to support that belief! Having been through so much disappointment as to render me emotionally numb, I just went on, caring for my son as was my duty, but wondering if this person and I were ever going to get along. It was a hard thing to think about after a long series of challenges, especially because for a long time my energy had been focused on every kind of survival rather than any kind of enjoyment.

It wasn't until years later that I realized I was not the only one who had experienced this. It *wasn't* because I was a single mother and didn't "have enough" to give to the baby. It *wasn't* because there was anything wrong with me or my son, and it *wasn't* anything to really worry about, so long as my son was well cared for and protected and I was taking care of my own needs for mental health. It wasn't colic, it wasn't neglect, and it wasn't a food allergy or any kind of disease (although those things need to be weeded out). I simply had a difficult baby. While some people will act as though a baby is difficult because you are doing something *wrong*, that is simply not true. Even my mother didn't believe it until we had one in our hands: Difficult babies exist.

As he grew, and as other children his age entered their terrible twos, my son was no longer the standout—but his healthy set of lungs and stubborn determination held on until he was almost five. In those years, we had been "fired" by three babysitters (although the caretakers at our eventually selected day care insisted that such people were obviously not professionals). When my son was four we traveled to England together, and I bought a children's chapter book about the Vikings for us to read on the plane. According to the book, in Viking society, the mother with the loudest, most badly behaved, and most dominant child would be well-respected in the community, as it was known that her child would be a great Viking! I wondered, "Why couldn't we have been Vikings?"

A happy conclusion to a potentially stress-inducing story: Difficult babies don't always turn into difficult adults. By the time my son was in kindergarten, he was a model citizen. Throughout elementary school, he was a perfect student. Now, as an adult, is a happy, healthy, functional and contributing member of society.

In conclusion, you too might have a difficult baby, although it's rare: I am the only one I knew who had these challenges, but have read some compassionate articles by others who have also had, and successfully raised, difficult babies. If you end up with a difficult baby, it's important not to feel like there's anything wrong with you or the child. You simply have the baby who would have been the best Viking—and you, his strong and well-respected mother, should be proud...

...and dedicated. According to a 2008 article posted on Psychology today by Jay Belsky, Ph.D., "One recent study shows that when infants who proved difficult and highly negative across their first six months of life are cared for in a warm, sensitively responsive manner by their mothers during their opening years of life, they show the least behavior problems and greatest social skill of all children as first graders. Just the opposite happens, though, with children with similar temperamental proclivities who experience insensitive care; they manifest the most problems and least social competence early in their school careers."

So if your baby earns you strange looks in public, "un-vitations" to birthday parties, or a "don't have room" from your local lazy babysitter, just know that you've got a special one because you're a special mom.

Bonding

Thankfully, despite my having a Viking baby, I had done one very important thing very right: My mom and I had diligently worked with my son to make sure he could see that life was full of love, happiness, and security, giving him the framework to be an emotionally healthy and bonded human being. It wasn't until many years after the birth of my son that I had known someone who had not properly bonded with his mother, and I learned the very sad consequence of attachment disorders.

I'd had *some* idea about attachments disorders at the time of my son's birth. My father had told me that orphaned babies whose physical needs for life were met but didn't have anyone holding them and loving them would die, and that this was the result of an experiment done in a crowded orphanage somewhere in Asia or Eastern Europe under

USSR occupation. But I had never considered the wide range of possibilities for babies who had experienced something in-between satisfactory interaction and fatal neglect.

Regardless of how you *feel* when your child is an infant, and regardless of whether your baby seems to *want* interaction, it is very important that you go through the motions of being 100 percent present in order for your baby to learn about human connections on a very fundamental level. This is easier to do if you breastfeed, but even if you don't, you can give your baby the proper interaction by talking to your baby, looking into his eyes, telling him stories, holding him, singing to him, dancing with him, and playing with him—and you can make up for long periods of time away—a work day or a visitation day, for example—by sleeping with your baby. Even if he doesn't "give back" or respond to show your efforts are working in any way, this early interaction may be what makes the difference between a healthy and functional adult and someone who suffers life-long depression and lacks a sense of belonging or connectedness.

Is it the Baby Blues, or is it Something More?

One reason why it's important to have someone in your home with you—if only intermittently—for the first six weeks of your motherhood is for the sake of observation. After you've had a baby, your hormones can go all out of whack. While a great many new mothers experience what's known as the Baby Blues, which includes mild depressive symptoms for the first few days to two weeks postpartum, one never knows whether those blues are going to be longer-term and are the beginning of postpartum depression. Having someone around who knows you well is a good opportunity to have someone to bounce things off of. They can observe whether or not you seem to be yourself, you can have honest discussions, and they can help ensure that you get much-needed food and rest which will diminish the likelihood of a false-positive self-diagnosis for postpartum depression.

If after two weeks you feel like you still feel consistently down or if you find yourself having fatalistic thoughts or moments of violent inspiration, you are likely suffering from postpartum depression. Many new mothers end up falling deeply into postpartum depression before they truly know what's going on. Postpartum depression is a hormonal condition that has nothing to do with whether or not you're a good person or a good mother. Single mothers are at a greater risk at developing postpartum depression because they normally have an increased workload and greater sole responsibility than partnered mothers, and exhaustion can affect a person's hormonal balance as well as other things. Get help as soon as possible if you feel like you are losing your ability to be happy or are about to do something violent or destructive to yourself, your family, or the baby.

While it's terrible to learn that despite everything you've done to keep yourself in great shape, you still need help, the good news is that help is in your own hands when you've learned to be your own best friend. If you are not breastfeeding, go straight to your grocery market and get some Saint John's Wort. Many studies have confirmed that Saint John's Wort is every bit as effective as taking Prozac to combat depression. It costs less than prescription medication, is easier on your liver, and doesn't require a doctor's approval. While opinions vary widely over whether it is safe to take while you are still pregnant or while breastfeeding (google the research and follow your instincts), if you fear or anticipate the onset of depression and are not breastfeeding, there is nothing wrong with taking it right away after the baby is born. The bad news is that it can take up to six weeks to take effect (so—my personal advice—commit to taking it as directed for at least nine weeks, and don't give up).

If you have insurance that covers mental and psychological health, the healthiest and most permanent way of combating postpartum depression is to train your brain to be happy through a combination of talk therapy and bio-feedback (also known as neuro-feedback). Your mental health professional will not only listen and affirm your right to feel the way you do, but will also conduct sessions in which he puts electrodes on your head and measures your brainwaves. After your current brainwaves are assessed, your counselor will give you exercises (in the form of video images) to help you to use the "happy" parts of your brain. You can tell if you're doing it right, because you will have an incentive project on the screen. For example, your screen may feature a closed rosebud. When you are using the correct parts of your brain, the rosebud will open. Your counselor will ask you to open the rosebud as many times and as quickly as you can by using your thoughts. After a while, your brain will exercise itself into being happy again.

Even if you don't have the right insurance, there may be a way for you to reap the benefits of bio feedback: There are computer-based bio-feedback "games" that feature the same exercises. However, with the computer games you don't get the benefit of supplemental talk therapy, and your benefit from this game will depend on your discipline and the regularity with which you play.

The main drawback of bio-feedback is that it does not reap immediate results. It takes up to six weeks of diligent practice in order to see a difference in your mental and emotional health, and six weeks can be a very long time for someone who is currently on the edge. However, if you stick to the program, bio-feedback can teach you such control over your emotions that you may never find yourself is a state of psychological emergency ever again, no matter what happens to you.

Despite the fact that you may want to do the absolute healthiest thing for your body, the unfortunate truth is that sometimes single mothers need help right away. The most immediate way to get results is to take an antidepressant or anti-anxiety medicine, which can be prescribed by your doctor, counselor, or nurse practitioner. However, taking drugs that completely change your brain chemistry can be extremely risky. Some of my friends who have taken anti-depressants had to try up to five prescriptions until they found one that made them feel better instead of worse, and there is always a certain amount of time one needs to "wean off" an anti-depressant. Do what you need to do in order to stay grounded, but listen to your body's reaction, and start your medication regimen under observation of a loved one if possible.

If you need immediate relief from depression, go to your doctor, nurse practitioner, or psychological counselor, and let them know you need help right away. If you don't have insurance, you will have to pay for this initial visit, but at the time of this writing, you can fill your subsequent prescriptions at your local Planned Parenthood office for a donation in an amount you can afford.

Don't feel guilty if certain plans fall through.
So you wanted to use cloth diapers because you just couldn't bear the thought of glutting the public landfills with non-biodegradable waste, and you wanted to breastfeed your baby and give her all the immunities that can only be acquired through her mother's milk, but you don't have enough time to haul all those diapers to the Laundromat, and the incision from your C-section hurts so badly that you can hardly sit up to breast feed your baby. *Relax.* If your plans must change, they must change. Do the best you can. If you have to abandon a past commitment, don't look at it as a failure. Instead, try to regard it as a special circumstance. It's nobody's business but your own, and (as we've discussed several times in this book) you have got to be your own best friend and refuse to judge yourself.

Allow yourself lots of time to prepare.
That first trip to the doctor's office is going to be a nerve-wracking experience, but it will get easier. Start getting ready to leave long before you normally would, just in case the baby decides to give you a hard time while you're dressing him, or in case you find that you don't know how to detach your car seat after all. Make sure you pack your diaper bag the night before so that you don't get stalled when everything else is going haywire. Leaving the house to tend to tasks will get easier as time goes by.

Take advantage of conveniences.
Make sure you know the locations of all the full-service gas stations in your area or bring a debit card or credit card so that you can pay at the pump rather than wonder if you should take your baby inside the gas station to pay or leave him in the car. Research the whereabouts of local drive-through restaurants, teller machines, and twenty-four hour supermarkets that can meet your needs on your very special schedule. Make sure your supermarket has carts with infant seats—you can't put many groceries in the cart if they're sharing space

with a car seat, and it will be hard enough to get organized and get to the grocery store once a week. Some cities have special parking spaces for new mothers. Find out if this is the case in your town, and get whatever permit you need in order to use them.

Get out of the house. NOW!!
Once you have a baby, it takes far longer to do just about everything. Sometimes new mothers think it's easier to stay around the house than to go through the hassle of packing everything up for a half-hour walk, but as any dog owner can tell you, even a half hour change of scenery can make a world of difference in the life of a dog—it's the same for a baby and a new mother. If you live in a temperate climate, take your baby for a walk. Go to the park, the museum, outdoor cafes, shopping, running errands, etc. Just being outside will help you feel connected with the outside world, and will be entertaining for the little one as well. If you live in a cold climate, bundle up your baby for a short walk, take your baby to the mall, or to visit friends and relatives. If your cold climate is also an icy one, invest in a good pair of ice cleats to put over your shoes so you don't slip, and get accustomed to them before the baby comes. Hire a babysitter or commission a trusted friends or relative to watch the baby for an evening and treat yourself to a night on the town every two weeks or so. When you do run errands, only do a few things at a time, doing what is most important first, and don't wait 'til the last minute. You may run out of steam quickly, and should not let yourself get exhausted. Stay away from germ-infested areas and people who are ill, and wash your hands frequently. Be careful, but not paranoid.

Beware the overly-eager suitor.
Single mothers are in a vulnerable situation: We may be in dire need of money, company, or someone to help us schlep our gear, and most of us feel that an enthusiastic partner would round out the picture nicely. However, *no* amount of money or help is worth compromising the safety and welfare of our children, and it is much better to be alone and free than in a bad situation. You must be extra cautious of the company you keep now that you have a child. Try to break into any relationship you have slowly, and keep a safe distance between your new suitor and your child until you have developed a very trusting relationship. Some men perceive that your standards might be lower due to your vulnerability and will try to muscle their way into your life. Some narcissistic men will flatter you like you never thought possible and you will become dependent on them, but then the tables will turn and they will start to devalue you and abandon you at the very worst time. Some men with dominance issues will shroud their dysfunction with what seem to be genuinely good intentions. Some men who are overly eager to be around you and your child are simply *pedophiles*, as demonstrated in Nabokov's *Lolita*.

Following are a few rules for being the vigilant single mom with high standards for the company she keeps:

Never allow yourself to appear desperate for money or a relationship. Don't complain to men (other than trusted friends) about being poor, lonely, or physically worn out, as this may indicate that you are desperate enough to allow yourself to be controlled. Although it may be hard to keep your mouth shut, don't complain about the baby's father either (women with "baggage" make for easy victims). If a man you think is interested (either reciprocated or not) asks about the baby's father, simply say that he's not involved in your life and change the subject. The details of what you've been through should be explored on *your* terms and only with someone you trust and know *very well*.

Do not accept lavish personal gifts from a man unless the attraction is mutual. Accepting his gifts may indicate a sort of "agreement" that he can court you, and it will be harder to get him out of your life unless the line is clearly drawn at your first opportunity. In addition, never use the concept of "timing" as an excuse not to date someone, because he may interpret this as his green light to bother you until the "time is right."

Be extremely cautious about any man who seems to be competing with your child. These characteristics can come in many forms, such as apathy towards you high standards of your child's care, a desire to take the attention away from your child, a tendency to distract you while you are performing important tasks, or a lack of attention to your baby's very clear signals.

Do not allow a suitor to criticize your parenting choices. You are this child's parent. If you end up marrying a man within the early years of your child's life and your child's father is not around, this man *may* become a father to your child. However, your current boyfriend has no right to make any judgments against the decisions that you make. He should simply be like a friend to your child: spoiling him, playing with him, and encouraging him, but he should not be allowed to (or even want to) discipline your child. Try not to rely on your boyfriends as baby sitters, because this is establishing a dependent relationship, which indicates that this man is in the running for a serious long-term relationship with you and your child.

Finally, *if the man who is interested in you has other children and does not pay child support,* **he is not the kind of man you want in your life!** It does not matter if you're prettier, smarter, nicer, or more stable than the mother of his children—if he's done it to her, *there's nothing to keep him from doing it to you!* Also, as a general rule, it is wise to stay away from a man who complains to no end about his past girlfriends, so take it as a warning sign if all a man wants to tell you is in connection with what he's had and doesn't want again. Your experience has given you the opportunity to learn a valuable lesson about life. If you heed only one piece of advice from me, let this be your primary lesson and learn it well: Don't repeat past mistakes!

Realize that things would not necessarily be any easier if you did have a partner.
Although it may seem as though married women and those who have partners active in their children's lives have a much easier time caring for their newborns than you do, the fact still remains that the majority of them don't have ideal situations either, even if things appear to be peachy keen on the outside. There are a great many men out there who still believe that raising children is the *sole* responsibility of the woman, and that includes feeding them, dressing them, changing them, entertaining them, waking up with them in the middle of the night, taking them to the grocery store, and even carrying them around, regardless of who's stronger or who has a more flexible schedule, and even who's earning the money! In many couples, especially those who are not married, the father of the child has stuck around out of a sense of obligation and does not truly want the child, the mother, or any of the responsibility of caring for either of them. Such a man is doomed to leave sooner or later. This may seem like a bit of a stretch, but you are actually at an advantage to these women because you've known where you've stood throughout this whole ordeal and have not been tied down to a relationship that is tepid or one-sided. At least you are not giving the best years of your life to someone who might just throw you away. You have your *freedom*! You can use it to be the sole foundation of your child's self-esteem and you can go out and get the job, the life, and the even man you want!

Get your child care arranged as soon as you can.
If you are going to need day care, research your options within the first weeks of your maternity leave, or possibly even while you are still pregnant. Depending on your income, you may qualify for Day Care Assistance (also called Child Care Assistance) or other special types of funding for your child care expenses (do an internet search that is specific to your state of residence). When you find a day care option you think you like, Interview the provider about her philosophies on discipline and schedules, take a look at the facility, and choose the one that makes you most comfortable and your child most welcome.

Remember to Eat!
Even if you are trying to lose weight, starving yourself will make you crazy much sooner than it will make you slim, and right now there are enough things trying your sanity to throw another risk factor on the pile.

During the first year of your child's life, you must have consistent access to healthy foods (that you like) that you can grab and eat on the run or turn into a meal at two o'clock in the morning if you have to. Always make sure your kitchen is stocked with the following items:

Granola bars/ Energy bars (or similar)

Eggs: Almost anything you make from scratch requires eggs. And as boring as it may be, a boiled egg can always serve as a snack that can take the edge off.

Bananas: Nutritionists say the banana is the perfect food. Babies like them too!

Fresh vegetables and dressing or dip: Always cut carrots, celery, and broccoli as soon as you get home from the store so you can grab and eat at a moment's notice. Salad dressing, yogurt dip, and hummus are great accompaniments.

Fresh fruit in season: Again, cut fruits like strawberries ASAP so you can eat quickly if you have to or bring them with you in a plastic container with a good seal.

Your favorite healthy breakfast cereal: If you are hungry and in need of fiber, bran cereal can serve double duty.

Powdered milk: It's never fun to run out of milk when you need it, and powdered milk takes a good long time to spoil.

Frozen vegetables: While which vegetables you have is a matter of taste, I always have peas and corn. If you have just a little bit of an entrée left over from the night before, vegetables can turn it into a meal.

Nuts: Nuts are a great source of protein when you don't have time to cook fish or meat, and some are high in Omega 3 fatty acids, which will keep your mood elevated.

A variety of teas, both with and without caffeine: The habit of drinking herbal tea throughout the day will keep you hydrated and will curb your tendency to reach for a soda.

Pasta and pasta sauce: This can always be combined to make a quick warm meal even if your energy is low.

Juice boxes: While juice boxes don't always provide a large enough serving to satisfy an adult, the boxes are lightweight, and a new mother who is carrying lots of gear doesn't need to lug around more heavy stuff than is necessary—and if drinking a small box of juice satiates the sugar craving steers you away from a soda, it's a win for you.

Canned soup and crackers: Canned soups are not the best food to eat every day, as many of them are high in sodium. However, if you have a favorite canned soup, make sure to have a couple of cans on hand. Always have your favorite crackers to go with cheese, soup, hummus, etc.

Dark chocolate: If you have a sweet tooth, dark chocolate is just about the best thing you can treat yourself to—it's high in antioxidants, and helps elevate your mood.

At least three instant meals, TV dinners, or frozen pizzas: Like with canned soups, Don't make a habit of eating only frozen meals because they are expensive and can be high in sodium and calories. But look for healthy alternatives and have a few on hand. Some highly organized moms and homemakers will make their own freezer meals—manicotti, chicken pot pie, soups, and casseroles—to keep in the freezer. As mentioned in the baby shower chapter, sometimes you can commission friends to bring home made freezer meals.

Canned tuna: Canned tuna is also high in mood-lightening Omega-3 fatty acids. Use Omega-3 mayonnaise, found in health foods section, to further help combat the blues. Add chopped celery, capers, dill, and a bit of cayenne to make it more exciting.

Your favorite cheese: If you like cheese and don't have a cheese slicer, now is the time to invest in one so you can minimize the time it takes you to get to that sanity-saving snack.

Clean water: While some people have no choice but to buy bottled water, filtered tap water is often just as safe, and can be carried in recycled or reusable bottles. While filters that attach to one's tap can be expensive, a filtering pitcher is generally affordable. Water used to make formula should always be filtered.

Vitamin Supplements: A daily multivitamin supplement should help your nutrition, even if you don't remember to take one every day.

When you leave your home, always be sure to bring a juice box, a granola bar (or similar), a small bottle of water, and a banana too (if you don't think it will squish) even if you only plan to be out for a short while. If you let yourself get too hungry, your patience with your baby and the world around you is sure to be thin.

When you do have time to have a real meal, make sure it is balanced. Eat meat, chips, and fried food in moderation, avoid fast food like it's your worst enemy (because it is). New mothers and working families can do well to invest in a crock pot: Turn it on in the morning, have dinner at night. If ever you are treated to a restaurant meal, eat the grilled wild (not farmed) salmon if it's an option, and keep in mind that rice and beans are a great healthy combination for protein. Also invest in a few Tupperware-type containers and save the leftovers from when you do make a real meal or go out to eat.

Eating is one of life's pleasures, but it's also one of life's necessities. If you get into the habit of addressing your need to eat with healthy foods that will positively affect your mood, you will greatly enjoy the opportunity to savor a good meal when you are able to sit and relax.

Epilogue

So, you have made it to the end of the book...

Did you by any chance notice anything different about this book from other pregnancy books you have read? I mean, aside from the fact that it is for *single* women—did you happen to notice that this book wasn't so much about the baby as it was about *you*?

That's right: This book was for *you*. Some authors, educators, and advocates subscribe to the idea that a pregnant woman/mother's entire purpose in life is to support the baby, that the baby is *more* important than its mother, so for a mother to want to strengthen herself and continue along her life path is selfish, reducing her purpose to that of a broodmare (this is particularly true for groups and organizations that promote infant adoption). While many women will feel the mother bear spirit or a profound attachment to the baby from the moment she conceives, to say that the baby is more important than the mother is like saying that a beautiful house does not need a strong foundation. The fact is that without a strong foundation, the house is not sound. You are the foundation, and it is a wiser investment to find the weak spots and repair them than it is to paint the trim in the guest bedroom.

Although I've tried to be thorough in preparing you for your experience as a new mother with an infant, everybody's experience is different. You may cruise through your pregnancy and new motherhood as though it were the most natural thing in the world for you to handle, and you may have such a tough time that the advice I've given in this book doesn't even begin to address your struggles.

Whatever your experience, I hope that giving you a heads-up of what you might encounter has made you more prepared and more confident that you can handle whatever comes your way.

I, for one, have confidence that you are going to turn out to be the very best mother any child could ever hope for and that you're not going to miss a step towards fulfilling your own personal hopes and dreams. I bet that within five years you are going to have a happy and healthy child, a beautiful and comfortable home, the job of your dreams (or at least a very good idea of what that is, as well as having laid some groundwork to get it), and that any man in your life is going to be a worthy partner who really loves and respects you for who you are. Your needs will be well met, which will give you control over your level of happiness. You will be in the habit of taking initiative and making changes when something is not right.

No matter what challenges you face in the immediate future, remember to take care of yourself in the moment, and don't let anything or anyone take the moment from you.

Eat healthy foods, exercise, learn all that you can, vote in every election, be frugal (but not stingy) with your money, stay focused on your dreams and know they are attainable, and keep your standards high. Love yourself.

I *know* you can do all of these things. I know this because I did them, and I didn't have a great helper like me taking me by the hand and showing me how it's done. I had to learn all this stuff the hard way, by going through it—and then later on, trying to help others, and then learning about what *they* went through. As a matter of fact, the learning process never ends. However, it is all a pleasure if I can take my experience and pass it on to help you be a happy and responsible person, a good mother, and the head of a very special family.

I am privileged in the event that this work has made a positive difference in your life and that of your beloved child.

Works Cited

(And some not cited)

The following books and movies added to my education in spirituality, nutrition, and social science, and were thus instrumental in helping me write *The Single Woman's Guide to a Happy Pregnancy*.

Books

Anderson, Margaret L. and Patricia Hill Collins. <u>Race, Class, and Gender: An Anthology.</u> Wadsworth: Albany, NY, 1998

Beeghley, Leonard. <u>The Structure of Social Stratification in the United States, Third Edition.</u> Allyn and Bacon: Needham Heights, MA, 2000

Hooks, Bell. <u>Feminism is for Everybody.</u> South End Press: Cambridge, MA, 2000

Khalsa, Dharma Singh M. D. <u>Food As Medicine.</u> Atria Books: New York, 2003

Nabokov, Vladmir. <u>Lolita.</u> Everyman: New York, 1992

Ore, Tracy E. <u>The Social Construction of Difference and Inequality: Race, Class, Gender, and Sexuality.</u> Mayfield: Mountain View, CA, 2000

Rampton, Sheldon and John Stauber. <u>Mad Cow USA.</u> Common Courage Press: Monroe, ME, 2004

Schlosser, Eric. <u>Fast Food Nation.</u> Houghton Mifflin: New York, 2001

Silverstein, Olga and Beth Rashbaum. <u>The Courage to Raise Good Men.</u> Penguin: New York, 1995

Walsch, Neale Donald. <u>Conversations With God, An Uncommon Dialogue Book 1.</u> G. P. Putnam's Sons: New York, 1996

Movies

Crucible, The. Dir. Nicholas Hytner. 20th Century Fox, 1996

Internal Affairs. Dir. Mike Figgis. Paramount, 1990

Purple Rain. Dir. Albert Magnoli. Warner Bros., 1984

Super Size Me. Dir. Morgan Spurlock. IDP, 2004.

Tie Me Up! Tie Me Down! Dir. Pedro Almodovar. Miramax, 1990

What the Bleep do We Know!?. Dir. William Arntz and Betsy Chase. Samuel Goldwyn/ Roadside Attractions, 2005.

Printed in Great Britain
by Amazon